THE COMPLETE MENOPAUSE HANDBOOK

Patricia Ann Featherstone

First published in Great Britain in 1993 by Carnell Limited,
37 Salisbury House, London Wall, London EC2M 5PJ.

Typeset by SJ Design and Publishing, Bromley, Kent.

Printed by Repro City Limited, London.

ISBN 1-85779-168-1

Belong To. R. E Roper.

Table of Contents

INTRODUCTION 5

WHAT IS THE MENOPAUSE? 9

It All Starts With Puberty . . . Hormone Production Is Reduced . . . Premenstrual Syndrome . . . When Menstruation Begins To Come To An End . . . When The Menopause Actually Occurs . . . The Early Menopause

SHORT-TERM SYMPTOMS OF THE MENOPAUSE 21

Hot Flushes . . . Night Sweats . . . Palpitations . . . Sleep Difficulties . . . Changes In Skin And Hair . . . Alterations In Menstrual Flow . . . Painful Periods

PSYCHOLOGICAL SYMPTOMS OF THE MENOPAUSE 34

The Empty Nest Syndrome . . . Evidence Of Aging . . . Health Problems . . . Work Problems . . . Changes In Sexual Patterns . . . Bereavements . . . Worrying About The Menopause . . . In Conclusion

DEPRESSION AND THE MENOPAUSE 44

SEXUALITY AND THE MENOPAUSE 53

GENITO-URINARY CHANGES DURING THE MENOPAUSE 63

Cystitis . . . Vaginal Thrush . . . Urinary Incontinence . . . The 'Squeeze' For Urge Incontinence . . . The 'Squeeze' For Stress Incontinence

OSTEOPOROSIS AND THE MENOPAUSE.................................75

The Link Between Osteoporosis And The Menopause . . . Predicting The Risk Of Bone Fracture . . . How Osteoporosis Can Be Prevented . . . Calcium And Nutrition

THE MENOPAUSE DOESN'T HAVE TO BE A MISERY...............83

Coping With Stress . . . Relaxation Techniques . . . Dealing With Insomnia . . . Physical Exercise . . . Sensible Dieting . . . Alcohol Intake . . . Looking Good

HOW OTHERS CAN HELP YOU...92

Your Family Doctor . . . Alternative Therapies . . . Self-Help Groups

HOW HORMONE REPLACEMENT THERAPY WORKS 102

SPECIAL ASPECTS OF HORMONE REPLACEMENT THERAPY 114

Pre-Existing Medical Conditions . . . What Screening Is Recommended? . . . Possible Side-Effects Of HRT . . . The Older Postmenopausal Woman . . . The Breast And Hormone Replacement Therapy . . . Prevention Of Breast Cancer . . . Contraception And Hormone Replacement Therapy

APPENDIX A – SOURCES OF HELP AND ADVICE 127

APPENDIX B – GLOSSARY 130

Introduction

At any given time something like ten million or more women in this country are affected by the menopause and the symptoms which precede and follow it. While many of these women will have a comparatively easy passage, many more will suffer all kinds of misery as their change of life takes place. As such, the menopause must rank as probably the largest single source of discomfort, stress, pain and worry, affecting the most people at a single moment in time.

If the menopause were a disease, it would be compared to a plague; but as it is a natural progression from one stage of life to another, its unpleasant side-effects are often largely ignored or passively accepted by many sufferers. Although modern medical science in recent years has come up with a wealth of treatments that can almost completely eradicate the negative effects of the menopause, only a very small percentage of women affected seek out and receive effective help. Yet the help is there . . . generally available just for the asking. Why then are so few benefiting from it?

The answer to that question is complex, involving as it does several distinct aspects. First of all, it could be said that women themselves can be their own worst enemies in this instance by being willing to put up with all kinds of symptoms – usually because they believe these to be 'natural' – without demanding that something should be done. Secondly, the medical profession, which should be the prime provider of both information and specific treatment, has itself a divergence of opinion about how to treat menopausal symptoms. This divergence reflects itself in the varying degrees of attention and assistance a woman might get when she consults her family doctor. Thirdly, the media has often played a negative role in the way they have reported scientific advances in menopausal management with 'scare stories' often obscuring and even distorting the facts.

The situation is generally further confused by two opposed views about the menopause:

- Its symptoms are the result of a hormone deficiency disease and this needs to be treated to ensure the health of women in later years; or
- It is a 'natural event' and women can deal with it on their own and there usually is no need for them to resort to medical help.

As is so often the case, both of these seemingly contradictory statements are true . . . *to an extent.*

To begin, let us look more carefully at the first statement. Yes, nearly all the menopausal symptoms are the result of hormone deficiency, but this is hardly a disease as this deficiency is one occurring naturally with the aging process. As far as the need to treat – or rather correct by replacement – this hormone deficiency is concerned, you can look at this in one of two ways. If the symptoms are severe, yes, treatment will alleviate them; if the symptoms are minimal, there may be no need to do so and therefore perhaps nature should be allowed to follow its course.

As far as the second statement is concerned, of course, the menopause is a natural event and, yes, many women do cope with it very well on their own without outside help. However, just because some women whose symptoms are mild don't need help, it doesn't mean that such help should not be offered and made available to others whose experience of the menopause is more traumatic. Even those women who have an easy time with the menopause may still suffer greatly from its potential after-effects, some of which will not manifest themselves until many years later when it is generally too late for treatment to be as effective as it might have been earlier.

There is one aspect of the menopause, however, upon which all authorities can agree: it is a highly individual experience and one to which no two women will respond in exactly the same way. It is this very individuality of response that can make it very difficult for the experts to state categorically what is the best thing to do, not that this difficulty necessarily stops them from telling others what they think is good for them.

In this book, I have sought to avoid such categorical advice and instead have chosen to take the simple course of presenting the facts that are available in a way that the reader can use them to choose her own course of action. And some of the decisions involved can be complicated indeed as the potential benefits have to be weighed carefully against possible risks.

One such major decision that will be faced by every woman as she approaches the menopause is whether or not to choose to take hormone replacement therapy – or HRT, as it is commonly known. This treatment can indeed work wonders for just about all aspects of the menopause, yet it is not suitable for all women and in some instances can create additional hazards. HRT, while to be recommended in the vast majority of cases, is not to be entered into lightly and the decision to start treatment should only be made after you've fully examined the relevant facts. While HRT needs to be prescribed by a doctor, the decision whether to take it should not be his or hers alone and is one that should be a joint one. After all, it is your body and it is you who will either gain the benefits or suffer the consequences.

While many menopausal symptoms can only be treated by a doctor, there are also other areas where sufferers can do a great deal to help themselves. A large part of this book has been devoted to that subject – such as simple, everyday things you can do to minimise night sweats, hot flushes, anxiety and many other unpleasant side-effects of the menopause.

Although controversy and disagreement about many aspects of the menopause are likely to continue for the time being, there are some key points from which every woman approaching her middle years should take comfort:

- There is no need to suffer unpleasant symptoms in silence. Help is available from various sources; it's up to you to seek it out and ensure that you get what you need.
- While there are many opposing points of view about certain treatments, there is also a broad consensus of opinion about many of them as you'll find out in this book. Find out the facts for yourself and then make your own decision with, if need be, the advice of your doctor.
- Osteoporosis – which every year brings about the deaths of thousands of women who have gone through the menopause – is largely a preventable disease, although it is important that preventative treatment should be begun as soon as possible to be fully effective.
- The menopause is not something to be feared or dreaded. It is just another stage in life, albeit a very important one, and how you will be affected by it will depend largely upon how you approach it in the first instance.
- A great deal of research is going on all the time into new and better ways of providing relief from both the short- and long-term symptoms of the menopause and every year new or improved treatments are becoming available. Overall, the outlook for women entering the menopause has never been better than it is today – and it will almost certainly be better still in years to come.

Finally, I must thank all the people who gave so generously of their time and expertise to help me with the research for this book. They are too many to acknowledge individually, but to each and every one of them I would like to extend my grateful and sincere thanks.

Patricia Ann Featherstone

1 What Is The Menopause?

Put at its very simplest, the menopause is the cessation of menstruation and is something that will happen sooner or later to every woman who lives long enough to reach that stage of her life.

There is another term that is used less frequently and that is the 'climacteric' which in many ways is perhaps the more satisfactory one, deriving as it does from a Greek phrase denoting a 'critical phase'. And, as most women who have experienced the menopause will agree, it is indeed a very critical time for them in many different ways.

Strictly speaking, however, there is a difference in meaning between the words 'menopause' and 'climacteric'. The *World Health Organisation* defines the menopause as 'the permanent cessation of menstruation resulting from loss of ovarian follicular activity' and the climacteric as 'the period immediately prior to the menopause and at least the first year after the menopause'.

In this book, for the sake of convenience and to match current everyday usage of the word, we shall generally use the word 'menopause' in its broadest sense to denote not just the cessation of menstruation but also what happens before and after the menopause itself. That is, after all, how the vast majority of women use and understand the word.

Before proceeding further, there are a few other words that also require definition:

Premenopausal: Defines that period of time when a woman is menstruating regularly.

Perimenopausal: When the woman's periods have started

to become irregular, but there has been menstruation within the past year.

Postmenopausal: When a woman hasn't had a period for at least one year.

Yet, despite all these very specific labels, there is one phrase in common usage – the 'change of life' – that has much to recommend itself, signifying as it does not just one event but a series of them that link together to transport a woman from one stage of her life to another. And while the medical and semi-medical terms automatically seem to place the stress on the physical, menstrual and hormonal alterations that are happening during that time, the 'change of life' carries with it much broader connotations, suggesting that apart from the physical changes there are others also taking place. That, of course, is very much the case because the menopausal experience can affect just about every aspect of a woman's well-being.

However, for the time being, we shall temporarily set aside all these definitions and use the word 'menopause' as a catch-all term to cover all the events that are linked to it.

But to grasp fully what happens during the menopause, it is essential to have a clear understanding of how things are before it happens. So, if the menopause essentially is marked by the end of menstruation, we must first of all look at how menstruation works before it comes to its end. Particular attention must be paid to the role hormones play in first of all starting up the menstrual cycle and then continuing it for some 35 or so years.

IT ALL STARTS WITH PUBERTY

As the menopause signals the end of menstruation, so its beginning is marked by puberty, a time when major changes are taking place in the young woman's body. The age at which puberty starts is highly variable, but may be said to fall roughly between eleven and fourteen years although earlier and later puberty is not uncommon.

Nearly all of the changes linked to puberty are triggered by hormones and the process that leads to puberty begins when the *hypothalamus* part of the brain causes the *pituitary gland* to release gonadotrophin hormones, in particular FSH – the *follicle-stimulating hormone* – and LH – the *luteinising hormone.* These hormones will in turn stimulate the ovaries, making it possible for them to start producing two more hormones – *oestrogen* and *progesterone*, both of which will then become major influences as they enter the bloodstream. Each of these two ovarian hormones has its specific role to play in these changes and the released oestrogen will affect the formation of breast tissue, affect how the body lays down fat, start the growth of both pubic and underarm hair, and also stimulate the apocrine glands – which are a special kind of sweat gland found near the vagina, anus, navel and nipples.

The other important task of oestrogen is to bring about a steady enlargement of the ovaries which, of course, are themselves also the source of oestrogen. As the ovaries grow, they produce more oestrogen. This additional oestrogen in turn causes yet more growth of the ovaries and this process stabilises after a period of time ranging from about one to two years when the ovaries have become big enough for egg production. Once this stage has been reached, the follicle-stimulating hormone and luteinising hormone – which, as you'll recall, started the whole process originally – will then cause ovulation to occur as an egg is released from the ovaries into the Fallopian tubes.

At the same time, the scar tissue left on the ovary when the egg was released starts to change and eventually becomes a very small yellow and pink gland – called the corpus luteum – which begins to manufacture progesterone whose job it is to alter the lining of the uterus by making it highly vascular with additional layers of cells so that it can best receive a fertilised egg should conception take place. At the same time the blood supply to the uterine lining is increased as part of the same preparatory process.

If conception does occur by a sperm fertilising an egg, the egg – now called a *zygote* – will undergo rapid cell division as it travels down the Fallopian tube into the uterus. There it will initially float free for some four to seven days absorbing nutriment from uterine secretions before finally adhering to the mucous lining of the uterus – the *endometrium* – in the process known as implantation.

However, if conception does not happen a completely different sequence of events is triggered from about the 24th day of the cycle onwards. The hypothalamus stems the flow of releasing hormone to the pituitary gland which then reduces the flow of the follicle-stimulating and luteinising hormones to the ovaries. This, in turn, causes the ovaries drastically to reduce their output of oestrogen resulting in a much lower blood flow to the uterus. This decreased blood flow causes cells to die and the uterine lining, which had been prepared to accept a zygote, is eventually shed thereby precipitating the menstrual flow.

The cycle of egg production which began with puberty will carry on year after year until the last mature eggs have been produced, usually some four hundred or so although it has been estimated that every woman is born with some 70,000 potential egg cells. However, of these many thousands, fewer than 500 will actually become mature eggs. In passing, it is interesting to note that unlike male sperm which are formed continuously throughout adult life, all potential egg cells are present in the woman's body from the time she was born herself.

Although the above is but a brief description of the many complex changes that take place in a woman's body during each menstrual cycle, it is clear how great a role is played in this by the various hormones involved. Not surprisingly, when that regular cycle, which had been taking place for some thirty-five years or so, starts to change with the onset of the menopause the consequences are far-reaching in many respects.

HORMONE PRODUCTION IS REDUCED

One of the key factors of the menopause is that the ovaries no longer produce the same quantities of oestrogen and progesterone, with the output of both hormones being severely reduced – not completely stopped, as some might have supposed. Additionally, there are other small sources of oestrogen in the body. For example, the androgen steroid androstanedione is converted into oestrone – a form of oestrogen – in the liver and in the fat tissues. Additionally, some oestrogen also comes from the adrenal glands located on top of the kidneys. These small sources, added to the reduced output from the menopausal ovaries, means that the oestrogen supply to the body is maintained but at such a low level that in most instances it is not enough to prevent menopausal symptoms and problems.

Incidentally, it is considered that this continuous reduced supply of oestrogen explains why there is so much difference in how women may react to the menopause. Although the ongoing supply is always small, it can vary greatly from person to person and these variations can mean that one woman who has a relatively substantial ongoing output may have few menopausal problems as compared with another whose ongoing production is small.

So far, we have considered the role of the ovarian hormones only in relation to the reproductive system. However, they also influence many other aspects of the body and these aspects will also, of course, be affected when the hormonal supply begins to reduce.

Here are just a few of the things that are not linked to reproduction but which oestrogen does normally:

1) Helps to maintain the health of the blood vessels by acting in conjunction with prostaglandins – which are hormone-like substances.
2) Maintains and controls the supply of collagen to the skin, thereby promoting elasticity and also affecting the thickness of the skin.
3) Affects the condition and thickness of the hair.

Progesterone, the second female hormone produced by the ovaries, equally performs several tasks that are not directly linked to reproduction but which affect the well-being of the whole body:

1) Improves the operation of the immune system by acting in concert with prostaglandins and immunoglobulins.

2) Helps the body in retaining water and salt at the correct levels.

Equally importantly, it has been shown that the ovarian hormones play a key role in influencing mood and that oestrogen helps bring about the optimistic and happy outlook that often marks the first two weeks of the menstrual cycle, while progesterone is credited with affecting the mood during the last two weeks of the cycle.

PREMENSTRUAL SYNDROME

Evidence of how ovarian hormone production can affect both mood and disposition is clearly found in the 'premenstrual syndrome' or PMS, as it is also known, which covers the often drastic changes that can occur just before menstruation, a time when there is a great imbalance between oestrogen and progesterone levels. And this hormonal imbalance can create all sorts of symptoms including, among many others: headache, backache, highly variable mood swings, depression, fatigue, insomnia, irritability, odd food cravings, skin problems, putting on weight.

As a woman approaches the menopause, the PMS symptoms often become more marked as the fluctuations in the hormonal balance become even wider. For example, progesterone production will become reduced as ovulation becomes less frequent, allowing the endometrium to build up rather than being shed regularly. And, as a result, when eventually there is enough progesterone to precipitate the shedding of the endometrium, the menstruation will be heavier. What's more, the reduced level of progesterone is also likely to make the periods become irregular and unpredictable as well as worsening any PMS symptoms that may have been experienced before and even cause these to appear for the first time.

Before bringing to an end this brief explanation of the roles of the various hormones, there is one more that should be mentioned and that is *testosterone* which, although being the primary male hormone, is also produced in minute quantities by both the ovaries and the adrenal glands in women. Generally, this testosterone has little effect, but its rate of production increases generally in post-menopausal women and if this increase is large enough there may be a tendency for the woman to lose some of her feminism and acquire additional facial and body hair.

WHEN MENSTRUATION BEGINS TO COME TO AN END

As menstruation is the result of the body shedding a uterine lining that is no longer needed because conception didn't take place, it follows logically that when no further mature eggs capable of being fertilised are being produced by the ovaries that the uterine lining will no longer need to be thickened in preparation for possible implantation. However, a woman's years of potential fertility don't generally come to an abrupt stop with every part of the reproductive system grinding to a simultaneous halt. What happens instead is a gradual slowing down of the various processes and this – called the perimenopausal cycle – begins much earlier than most women believe, perhaps from the age of 35 onwards, and will generally be well underway by the age of 40.

However, although the menopausal process will have begun with great variations already taking place in the levels of various hormones, the woman in her late thirties or early forties will generally have little inkling of what is happening. This is because all of the outward signs will remain much the same with the menstrual periods probably remaining regular and no menopausal symptoms manifesting themselves.

But, as time progresses, changes will become apparent, the most immediately noticeable of these likely to be an alteration in the volume of the menstrual flow which may at times be either heavier or lighter than previously. This is, of course, the result of variations in the thickness – and therefore the amount – of the uterine lining which is being shed.

Conception still remains technically possible at this stage, although becoming more and more unlikely, so contraceptive measures, if required, must be continued.

Apart from changes in the menstrual flow, there may be few other symptoms in the early years of the perimenopause because the ovaries continue to produce oestrogen at just about the same level as before. This, of course, means that those symptoms linked to oestrogen deficiency – such as hot flushes, tiredness, vaginal dryness and so on – will not have started appearing as there is as yet no oestrogen deficiency, merely a steadily declining supply.

WHEN THE MENOPAUSE ACTUALLY OCCURS

Gradually the length of time between periods is likely to become more and more erratic with some periods perhaps being missed completely until there comes a time when there has been no bleeding for a year – and that stage is the point in time that traditionally is used to indicate that the menopause has been reached. Going back to the definitions at the beginning of this chapter, a perimenopausal woman is one whose periods have started to become irregular, but there has been at least one within the previous year; a postmenopausal woman is one who hasn't had a period for at least a year. So, according to the textbook definition, the menopause takes place at that very instant when a woman hasn't had a period for a year because up to that moment she is technically perimenopausal.

And it follows from the above that this hypothetical woman becomes postmenopausal just as soon as she has ceased being perimenopausal. One could take this reasoning somewhat further by suggesting that therefore there is no such thing as the 'menopausal' woman because by definition she is either *peri* or *post*menopausal, either having had or not having had a period within the past twelve months!

Of course, this reasoning, while technically correct, is a nonsense as everyone knows that the word 'menopause' is used to describe a whole series of events taking place over a lengthy period of time and not just a brief theoretical divide between two stages.

However, this theoretical measure does have one very practical use and that is to act as a yardstick by which the point at which a woman reaches the menopause can be calculated. There are numerous statistics available on this which show that – on average – the menopause occurs at the age of 50. However, a better way to put this is to say that it is most likely to happen between the ages of 49 and 51 and may take place quite normally between the ages of 45 and 54 and even between the ages of 40 and 60. Incidentally, the timing of the menopause is remarkably consistent throughout the world although there are some variations on a national basis. For example, the average age for the menopause in the United States has been calculated as being 51.4 years whereas in Great Britain it is 49.75 years. The same statistics also show that the menopause is likely to happen about two years earlier for women who are cigarette smokers or those who have undergone a hysterectomy that did not include the removal of the ovaries.

The age ranges above, of course, refer to 'normal' menopauses, although some women may stop menstruating in their thirties. These menopauses are considered premature and often occur abruptly without being accompanied by a clearly identifiable perimenopausal stage. Doctors still don't know what causes these premature menopauses which occur as the egg cells within the ovaries disappear spontaneously.

There are other reasons, of course, why menstruation may stop at an early age and these include the surgical removal of a woman's ovaries or damage done to them by irradiation. When the egg cells are destroyed in this fashion, the menopause will start suddenly and will be accompanied by the usual menopausal symptoms.

Apart from the broad indications above, it is almost impossible to predict when the menopause will happen in a specific case. Medical researchers have tried to establish databases to correlate the timing of the menopause with various other factors, such as the age at which menstruation began, whether the woman had had children and her age at the last birth, whether oral contraceptives were used and the number of pregnancies. However, by far and large, this research has failed to come up with any consistent results so there is little that can be said with certainty.

One factor, however, did emerge and that is that a woman can often get an indication as to when her menopause may occur by looking at the experiences of close blood relations – such as her mother, sisters, aunts, grandmothers – for it has been found beyond dispute that there frequently is a great similarity in timing within family groups.

THE EARLY MENOPAUSE

Whether a comparatively early menopause is a blessing or not depends very much upon the individual point of view as some women may welcome the ending of their menstrual cycle while others see themselves as being catapulted prematurely into a different stage of life – and one for which they feel they are not yet quite ready.

In some instances, if the end of the fertile years comes sooner than expected, this may also mean the abandonment of any hopes of adding further children to the family. And, somewhat perversely, it has been found that in some cases, the mere fact of becoming unable to have a child may make a woman wish that she could, even if she had shown no inclination in that direction before. It's as if the door closing on the possibility of childbirth makes the woman wonder whether perhaps she should have had a baby while she still had the chance.

One concern that is shared by almost all women as they reach the menopause – whether prematurely or not – is how they will cope with the various physical changes that are taking place and to what extent these changes are likely to affect their health, looks and general lifestyles. Additionally, they will be concerned at how long the transition through the menopausal years may take and to what extent they will be affected by the various symptoms they have heard about.

The length of the menopause – and here the term is used in its broadest sense – is highly variable from woman to woman, but it can be safely said that it usually takes at least two years and up to five from when the first changes in the menstrual cycle become noticeable until a woman experiences the last of the short-term symptoms. This, of course, is only a very rough guide as some lucky women seem to glide gracefully through the whole experience in a matter of months while for some others the problems that the menopause can engender will manifest themselves for much longer than five years.

Apart from the great variation in the length of time that the menopause takes, there are equally great variations in how much an individual woman may be affected by the experience. While all menopausal women undergo great fluctuations in hormone levels, the extent to which this affects them is by no means the same. Once again, a great deal of research has been done to try to pin down what a particular woman's experience of the menopause is likely to be and, again, many of the findings have been contradictory. Two factors, however, can serve as a guide:

1) A woman may be able to make a shrewd guess as to what she might expect by looking at the experiences of near blood relatives as her own pattern is quite likely to be a similar one.
2) Women often find that their menopausal process is much as they might have expected it to be before it actually started. In other words, if a woman believes beforehand that her menopause is likely to be an easy one, then the chances are greater that it will be so. On the other hand, the woman who dreads the oncoming of the menopause and fully expects to suffer from its attendant symptoms for years is more likely to find that her experience is indeed a particularly unpleasant one.

The above, of course, are generalities only and may or may not hold true in any particular case. About the only thing that can be said with anything approaching near certainty is that no two women ever experience absolutely identical menopauses because even if the hormone fluctuations are identical and the length, severity and incidence of the side-effects are the same, the women's own particular outlook and reactions to these will vary greatly.

One other factor that has emerged from the various studies is that the more knowledgeable a woman is about the menopause and the help available to combat its various symptoms, the more likely she is to be able to go through it with comparative ease. Knowledge – and making the correct use of it – is indeed a woman's most powerful ally in ensuring that her passage from one stage of life to the next one is as smooth and trouble-free as it can be. This must not be taken to mean that all the troublesome and worrisome aspects of the menopause can be eliminated, but that they can certainly be controlled and contained to a very great extent. How to achieve this is what the rest of this book is all about as in its chapters you will find out exactly what causes the various physical and psychological symptoms of the menopause and what you can do to minimise these in various ways.

While no one can promise you a menopause that will be completely trouble-free, there is no doubt that you can do a great deal to help yourself, by your own actions and reactions and by making the fullest use of all the assistance and support that is available nowadays from medical and other sources. As you read on, you will discover that the menopause doesn't have to be something that must be approached with dread as to its consequences, but perhaps merely a stagepost in your life, albeit a very important one.

2 Short-Term Symptoms Of The Menopause

Apart from the major changes that are taking place in the woman's reproductive system in the years preceding the menopause, most women will also experience several other connected symptoms.

Some of these symptoms will be obviously physical ones while others might be classified as being psychological. However, the dividing line between these two groups can be rather blurred as the so-called psychological symptoms are almost invariably due to a physical cause linked to the menopause itself.

Incidentally, the word 'symptom' is used throughout this book in its broadest sense – which is how the word is commonly understood by most people. Strictly speaking, according to the medical fraternity, a symptom is something of which the patient is aware herself such as, for example, hot flushes. On the other hand, doctors use the word 'sign' to denote something of which the patient is not aware and which is revealed either during a medical examination or subsequent tests, such as, say, a change in hormonal levels or blood pressure.

In other words, a patient might present herself to her doctor and complain of various 'symptoms'; the doctor's examination might then identify connected 'signs' and a diagnosis will be made on the basis of both symptoms and signs. So the symptom that a patient presents might be attacks of giddiness and the sign that the doctor discovers might be raised blood pressure. Useful though this distinction can be to the medical profession, it is ignored in this book and 'symptoms' will be used to describe both 'symptoms' and what might otherwise have been called 'signs'.

Before looking individually in greater detail at the various physical symptoms that may accompany the menopause, we will begin by listing some of the more common ones and these include:

- Hot flushes.
- Night sweats.
- Palpitations.
- Sleep difficulties.
- Changes in the skin and hair.
- Alterations in menstrual flow.
- Painful periods.

Additionally, there are many other symptoms that may accompany the menopause, such as sexual and urinary problems, putting on weight, changes in the structure of the bones and so on, but these will be dealt with in later chapters.

It is impossible to predict to what extent an individual woman may be affected by these symptoms as she enters her menopausal years. Surveys conducted both in Great Britain and the United States show that a small percentage of women – about 15 per cent – will have virtually no symptoms. On the other hand, ten per cent of women will report what they describe as 'severe' or even 'very severe' problems. These two figures, of course, indicate that about 75 per cent of all women will have some troublesome symptoms in varying degrees of severity.

The same surveys also showed that the symptom which was most widely reported was hot flushes, followed closely by night sweats and palpitations.

Useful and interesting that the statistical evidence resulting from surveys can be, it remains the case that it is but of little comfort for a woman who is having severe menopausal problems to learn that she is in a comparative minority. If there is one thing that just about all women who have been interviewed by researchers have agreed upon it is that the menopause is an intensely personal and individual experience. "You'd have to experience it yourself to understand exactly how I feel", is the phrase that cropped up time and time again in different forms as women found it almost impossible to communicate clearly to others exactly how they felt.

As we now proceed to look in detail at various symptoms, it's worth keeping the above in mind and understanding that while it may be possible to classify and describe symptoms, it is much more difficult to relate exactly how they may affect those who actually experience them.

HOT FLUSHES

While hot flushes – which, incidentally, are known as hot 'flashes' in the United States – are the most commonly complained of symptom, they are by no means universal and, depending upon which authority you choose to consult, occur in as many as 85 per cent to as few as just over half of menopausal women.

Doctors don't know exactly what causes these flushes, but the most likely explanation is that they are the result of a breakdown in the temperature control of the body which is governed by the *hypothalamus* of the brain. Under normal circumstances, the hypothalamus sends out nerve impulses along the autonomous nervous system to control regulatory mechanisms in the body to compensate for overheating or overcooling resulting from either heat gain or loss. It is believed that the decline in oestrogen during the menopause upsets this delicate mechanism and causes the sympathetic nervous system to dilate the blood vessels.

This dilation effect is known as '*vasodilation*' and means that some of the arterioles below the epidermis become wider and thereby cause a greater flow of blood near the surface. This, of course, means that there is an accompanying increase in the loss of heat through the epidermis by convection and radiation into the air.

The flushing – or reddening of the skin – is the directly visible result of the increased amount of blood flowing just below the epidermis and is, naturally enough, most visible in people who have fair skin.

The medical profession places hot flushes in the '*vasomotor*' category of symptoms, meaning that they are the result of changes in the size of the blood vessels. Generally, vasomotor symptoms – which also include night sweats and palpitations – are found to be most severe towards the end of the perimenopause and shortly afterwards, gradually reducing in frequency and severity as hormone production stabilises at new levels.

As to how frequently hot flushes may occur, there is a great deal of variation, as was found in one survey on the subject with roughly half the women interviewed (which only included those who had hot flushes) saying that they had one less than once a week. Twenty per cent said that they had them 'several times' a day while another 20 per cent said that they had them at least once a day. Ten per cent of the women said that the flushes occurred only once or twice a week.

Equally variable was the women's response to the question "Do you find the hot flushes distressing?" About half said that they didn't find them very distressing at all; another quarter found that they were distressing 'sometimes'; with about 15 per cent calling them 'not at all distressing' and just over ten per cent reporting the hot flushes as 'definitely distressing'.

How women themselves describe their hot flushes gives an indication of how variable the symptom may be:

"I have my hot flushes in batches. Sometimes I won't have any for several weeks and then – suddenly and for no particular reason that I can discern – I may have half a dozen or so within a couple of hours."

"When a flush starts, it's like my skin is being set on fire from the waist upwards until all of my upper body feels hot."

"The hot flushes are bad enough, but the sweating that goes with them is ten times worse. On a bad day I have to change clothes about six times."

"Yes, I've had the occasional hot flush, but maybe only about ten or so during the last year. I can't say that they bother me very much."

"It's very strange because I'm not really aware of it when I'm having one, although I've been told that I go all red in the face."

"I had the occasional hot flush before my menopause started. I can't say that things are all that different now."

While hot flushes may be disconcerting, distressing and at times perhaps embarrassing, they are not dangerous and are just one of the many normal side-effects of the hormonal changes happening during the menopause. Hot flushes can be controlled by Hormone Replacement Therapy – or HRT, for short. What this therapy is and how it works to reduce and even eliminate many of the unpleasant aspects of the menopause will be covered in full detail later in this book. However, apart from HRT – which is not suitable for or necessarily wanted by every woman – there are several practical things that you can do to help yourself:

- Cut down your intake of stimulants – including coffee, tea, alcohol and spicy foods – as these have been found to trigger hot flushes.
- Wear lightweight clothing, preferably made of cotton rather than artificial fibres. And, when the weather is cold, choose to wear several light layers of clothing rather than fewer but thicker ones as that way you'll be able to remove one or more layers if you start feeling too hot because of a flush.
- Don't try to fight a hot flush if you feel one coming on because you won't succeed in making it go away and the stress of trying to do so is only likely to make matters worse. Instead, try to relax and 'go with the flow'.
- Try to avoid stuffy, over-heated rooms.
- If you can, stop or cut down smoking as this increases your propensity to sweat. Sugar has somewhat the same effect, so cut down on that as well.
- When you're having a hot flush, you may be able to reduce its intensity and duration by standing near an open window. A cold shower, although obviously not always practicable, will help a great deal and, failing that, you might try running some cold water over your wrists.

NIGHT SWEATS

In many ways very similar to the hot flushes dealt with above are the night sweats that are experienced by many women during the menopause. Once again, night sweats are a vasomotor symptom and, like hot flushes, they are considered to be the result of changing hormone levels affecting the performance of the hypothalamus as it controls body temperature by dilating or constricting blood vessels.

Under normal conditions, a person starts to sweat, depending upon the clothing worn and activity engaged in, to reduce body temperature when the external temperature is above the range of 29 to 31 degrees Centigrade. Below this range, vasodilation of the arterioles is usually sufficient to keep the body cool enough. However, when the temperature of the blood reaching the hypothalamus is between half to one degree Centigrade above 'normal' – for whatever reason this might have happened – nerve impulses will be sent from it to stimulate the sweat glands into action. These glands will then draw fluid from the blood and pass this through minute ducts onto the surface of the skin. As the sweat evaporates in the air it takes with it latent heat from the body and thereby reduces the internal temperature.

Sweating therefore is the natural way for the body to restore its normal temperature. Night sweats, however, occur when there seems to be no need for the body to lower its temperature and are judged to be the result of faulty or incorrect signals received by the sweat glands. By the way, it's worth noting that sweat evaporation for temperature control is mainly from the forehead, neck, upper lip, face and trunk, while sweating from the armpits, soles and palms seems to be more dependent upon emotional stress or other psychological factors than on the needs of internal temperature control.

Not surprisingly, it has been found that women who have lots of hot flushes also have more night sweats. And, once again, their reaction to them varied a great deal:

"I don't mind the hot flushes; it's the night sweats that make life unbearable right now. There's nothing worse than waking up in the middle of the night lying in a bed that's soaked with your own sweat."

"I don't get any sleep at all some nights – if I'm not having any night sweats, then I lie awake worrying about whether I'm going to have them."

"Yes, I think that I've had a couple of bouts of night-sweating during my menopause, but I can't say that they were all that uncomfortable."

"There are times when I dread the very idea of going to bed as I know that I'll wake up soaking wet several times during the night."

"It's not so much the sweating at night that bothers me, but rather the shivering from the cold afterwards. And, of course, the lack of sleep is making my days miserable as well."

Although once again HRT will generally ease night sweating, there are also several simple measures you can adopt to make it easier to cope with the misery that it can cause:

- Use bedsheets made of cotton as they will absorb the moisture better.
- If the bedroom is on the cool side and you need bedclothes for warmth, then use several thin layers rather than one thick one. That way, should you have a night sweat, you can shed some of the layers while still retaining enough to stop you from shivering.
- If you're woken by a night sweat, don't panic. Try to relax, perhaps read for a while, without worrying too much about the sleep that you're missing.
- As advised for avoiding hot flushes, it may be useful to cut down on stimulants as well as smoking.
- Some women say that having a drink of water shortly before bedtime lessens the likelihood of night sweats. Others claim that keeping a window open has also helped.

PALPITATIONS

Distressing though palpitations can be, they are generally just one more symptom caused by the sympathetic nervous system as it responds to messages received from the hypothalamus. As we have seen before in the instances of other vasomotor symptoms, this temperature control works by dilating the blood vessels and this, in turn, is likely to give rise to an increased heartbeat rate and so produce the palpitations.

As a generality it can be said that palpitations should not be a cause for concern for the patient and that they certainly do not necessarily mean that she is having cardiac problems. However, there is no question that for some women a bout of palpitations can be a scaring experience, especially if they've never had them before, as proven by the following quotes:

"I felt as though my heart was racing and trying to break out of my chest. I don't mind admitting that it scared the hell out of me."

"When I had my first palpitations, I was quite certain that it was a heart attack. I remember thinking at the time that it was bad enough to be going through the menopause without having this as well."

"It's one thing to be told that palpitations aren't harmful and that the less notice you take of them, the sooner they will go away. It's quite another actually to have them ..."

The main medical answer to palpitations is once again HRT, although relaxation techniques and certain diet restrictions – which are covered in later chapters – may help you cope with them and perhaps also reduce the number of times you may have them.

While, as stated above, palpitations are a 'normal' part of the menopausal pattern for many women, you should never take it for granted that this is the case. If you have the slightest doubts at all you should bring them to the attention of your doctor so that he can eliminate any other possible causes.

SLEEP DIFFICULTIES

'Moderate to very severe' disturbances in sleep patterns were reported by 32 per cent of menopausal women interviewed in one recent UK survey and this figure is also supported by other surveys which came up with broadly similar findings.

However, although it is clear that the menopause is often marked by poor sleep patterns, many experts feel that the insomnia is not necessarily a direct result of the menopause itself, but perhaps quite often something that just also seems to happen around the same time of life.

"Most of us are troubled with indifferent sleep at one time or another," explained one doctor. "And any time that a person is under unusual stress one of the first things that often happens is that the quality and quantity of sleep goes by the board. The late forties and early fifties can be a difficult age for anyone, not just women who are going through the menopause, and it has also been found that men in that age group are equally likely to experience disturbed sleep patterns.

"It is likely, therefore, that much of the insomnia that is attributed to the menopause may not be the direct result of it, but rather comes about because the sufferer is at a stage of life where the worries just seem to pile up, perhaps because of physical signs of aging as well as ever-encroaching thoughts about a future that may seem uncertain."

So it follows from this that it can be quite important to try to identify and separate the reasons why sleep may be affected during the menopause. If the lack of sleep is the result, for example, of being frequently woken by night sweats, then it's clearly part and parcel of the menopausal symptoms and may also respond favourably to HRT. But if the insomnia is brought about by everyday worries that keep the sufferer from going off to sleep, then HRT is not likely to be of great help. Naturally enough, of course, whether or not the insomnia is linked to the menopause, there are several practical things you can do to make matters better and these will be dealt with later in this book.

Of course, the question as to whether the insomnia is caused by the menopause or not becomes rather difficult to answer if what is keeping you awake is worrying about the menopause! And, perhaps not unsurprisingly, that is what seems to happen quite frequently and is rather like the wryly funny but often quite true explanation given by some insomniacs: "I'm sure that I would sleep quite well if it wasn't for the fact that I lie awake worrying about my insomnia." This is not meant to suggest that insomnia is either a laughing matter or that 'it is all in the mind', but instead to underline the fact that the reasons for poor sleep are many and varied.

Incidentally, it is worth noting in this context that the Department of Health has recently advised family doctors to treat complaints about insomnia – and not just those linked to the menopause – somewhat more seriously than they might have done in the past. Lack of sleep may not be a serious medical condition, the Department noted, but the effect of it upon sufferers can be quite devastating and debilitating.

CHANGES IN SKIN AND HAIR

One of the things that women often worry about greatly as the menopause approaches is how it may affect their looks in general and, in particular, the condition and appearance of their skin and hair.

There is no question indeed that falling oestrogen levels will cause major changes in skin structure. What happens is that the skin collagen – which provides a major part of the connective tissues of the skin and helps support it – is lost at a much faster rate as the oestrogen drops. In fact, it has been estimated that as much as 30 per cent of the collagen may be lost in the ten years that follow the menopause itself.

The direct result of this collagen loss is skin that becomes gradually thinner and thinner as well as drier and which is more likely to show the effects of bruising. Additionally, the skin will also take on a slightly transparent and somewhat waxy appearance while wrinkles will increase in number as well as becoming deeper and more noticeable. Brown marks, also known as age spots, are also quite likely to make their first appearance around this time.

Not all women will experience these changes in the skin to the same extent and some lucky ones will almost appear to escape altogether these unpleasant side-effects of the menopause. Nevertheless, for the vast majority of women, a deteriorating skin remains a major concern as it is such an obviously visible sign of aging.

While these changes in the structure of the skin are perhaps not meaningful as far as the overall health of the patient are concerned, they are nevertheless often particularly feared – and even strongly resented – by women who not unreasonably wish to preserve an attractive, youthful appearance for as long as they can possibly do so. Skin creams and other moisturisers may help quite a lot in the early stages of change, but these will essentially only disguise or postpone what is slowly but inexorably taking place. HRT can provide a more lasting solution to the problem as it has been found that in six months or so it can bring back the lost collagen to the point it was at before the menopause began. Acting through the oestrogen receptors in the fibroblast cells – which develop the skin connective tissue – HRT will increase blood flow in the skin and also raise its water content, thereby making it more elastic and thicker to give it a more youthful appearance.

It is not quite so clear why the hair may be affected by the menopause except that its roots are deep in the skin connective tissue where the lower oestrogen levels bring about loss of collagen. But, whatever the exact mechanism causing it may be, many women report that their hair starts to become thinner as they enter the menopause. Whether this thinning is truly a by-product of the menopause is somewhat open to question as HRT, while being credited by some experts with improving hair condition, has not been proven conclusively to do so, although the argument about its efficacy in this instance continues until better evidence comes to light.

ALTERATIONS IN MENSTRUAL FLOW

As might be expected, one of the most common symptoms of the menopause are changes in the menstrual flow and this may be altered quite drastically in both its volume and duration. This variation in the pattern of menstruation may manifest itself in many different forms and is likely to affect something like up to 85 per cent of menopausal women. How variable the extent of these changes – and the way in which they manifest themselves – is reflected in what some of the women interviewed in one survey had to say:

"It seems as though my life has become one continuous long period – just as one finishes, I feel that I'm already getting the warning signs that the next one is due."

"My periods used to be as regular as clockwork and then the clock broke down completely and I wouldn't know from one day to the next whether I'd be having a period or not."

"I went for eleven months without a period and was sure that I had passed the menopause. Then, on the twelfth month, there was a bleed and I had to start the whole countdown all over again."

"My periods stayed much the same throughout, except for the last couple of months when they were about six weeks apart instead of the usual four."

Apart from the variations in the menstruation pattern, there are also frequently changes in the volume of the flow which can become either much heavier than previously experienced or alternatively can also become relatively scanty. While these changes, be they in the frequency of the periods or the menstrual flow, are quite normal during the perimenopause, it must be stressed that irregular bleeding is not and that any unexplained bleeding – such as between periods, after intercourse, or after the menopause has taken place – should be reported to your doctor for investigation.

In fact, the best advice is that if you entertain even the slightest doubt as to whether any bleeding is part of a 'normal' menopausal pattern or not, you should bring it to the attention of your doctor. Even if he finds that everything is as it should be, he may still be able to offer other help to control the problem.

PAINFUL PERIODS

Another common complaint associated with the menopause is that the periods may become more uncomfortable and even painful. Although this can once again be part of a perfectly normal pattern and is experienced by up to ten per cent of women, it too warrants you seeing your doctor.

The reasons for '*dysmenorrhoea*' – the medical name for pain that accompanies normal or abnormal menstrual bleeding – can be many and could include infection, fibroids or endometriosis, the latter being a condition in which small amounts of endometrial tissue are found outside the uterus itself such as on the ovaries or in areas between the rectum and uterus. However, whatever the cause might be, periods that have become painful are a matter for medical investigation and you should not hesitate to see your doctor about them.

Although the above includes most of the short-term physical symptoms associated with the menopause, there are others which are experienced less frequently and these will be examined later in this book. In the next chapter we will turn our attention to the so-called 'psychological' symptoms of the menopause.

3 Psychological Symptoms Of The Menopause

Apart from the clearly identifiable physical symptoms covered in the previous chapter, there are numerous other symptoms associated with the menopause. And the word 'associated' is used advisedly because there is a great deal of controversy as to whether some of these symptoms are indeed genuinely part of the menopausal process. There will be more about this later, but in the meantime, here's a list of the main so-called 'psychological' symptoms that for many women often form part of the menopause: swings in mood, irritability, anxiety, feelings of inadequacy, loss of energy, memory failure, lack of concentration, tiredness, weepiness and depression.

It's a formidable list and one that could make any woman facing the menopause fearful indeed of what awaits her. There are, however, two major points to be kept in mind: first of all, most menopausal women only experience some – if any – of these symptoms; and secondly, if they do, it's usually in quite a mild form that comes and goes at various times.

So, being menopausal doesn't mean that you're going to have to suffer any of the above – you may or you may not, depending upon your disposition and circumstances. And should you be among the unlucky ones who find that the menopause is also a time of phychological stress, the odds are that the manifestations of this will be fleeting and will probably disappear of their own accord in due course.

Before looking at the specifics of these various psychological symptoms in greater depth, we will return to the question of whether they are truly part of the menopause. The answer to this comes in two parts:

1) There is no question at all that a much greater incidence of these psychological symptoms is reported by menopausal women as proven by survey after survey. The medical profession as a whole accepts that these symptoms are part of the menopausal years for many women. So, on that basis alone, these symptoms can be fairly described as being part of the menopause, although not necessarily caused by it.
2) Broadly speaking, the medical profession admits it doesn't know for certain whether this increase in psychological symptoms is primarily due to the physical changes taking place during the menopause or is the consequence of other factors.

Putting it another, simpler way, no one is sure at this stage what causes these symptoms to appear with greater frequency during the menopause. However, much research – all of it so far less than conclusive - is being carried out to try to link cause and effect and determine once and for all whether the changes in hormonal levels actually cause or precipitate these symptoms.

There is, of course, a great deal of evidence from various sources about causation, but the trouble with this evidence is that it can point in opposite directions and you have to decide for yourself which findings you prefer to accept. For example, an article in the *Journal of the Royal College of General Practitioners* (J Coope, Is oestrogen therapy effective in the treatment of menopausal depression?) reported that oestrogen levels were not found to be lower in menopausal women who were depressed than in those who were not. On the other hand, a report in the *South African Medical Journal* (W H Utian, The mental tonic effect of oestrogens administered to oophorectomised females) concluded that oestrogen therapy had been found to have a marked beneficial effect on women's moods and acted as a 'mental tonic'. These are not the only examples of rather contradictory findings as medical literature abounds with them.

Although it will no doubt be useful eventually to find out what causes the symptoms to appear in the first instance, as that may point the way to preventing them, causation remains a somewhat academic point as far as sufferers are concerned in the meantime. And there usually is no question in their minds that their psychological symptoms are not only part of but also caused by the menopause.

Here's what some women had to say on the subject:

"I have always had what you might call a bright and happy outlook on life in general – that is until my change began and suddenly I became a very pessimistic person indeed who could only see the negative side of things."

"Ever since my periods have gone all funny, it seems as though my mind has gone the same way. I forget the simplest things and just can't seem to concentrate on anything for any length of time at all."

"My mood seems to change completely for no reason at all. One minute, I'm as happy as a lark; the next, I'm deep down in the blues."

"I'm just not very interested in anything and all I want to do is to mope around the house. I've tried to force myself to show an interest in various things and projects, but it just doesn't work."

"I used to take my job very seriously and took pride in being good at it. Now, although I'm managing to hang on to it, I really couldn't care less. I wouldn't be surprised if my employers were to let me go. What's more, I find it difficult to care too much either way."

"There is only one word to describe how I feel most of the time and that is 'inadequate'. I find it almost impossible to bring myself to do anything and when I do I just know that it's not going to work out right."

It's clear from the quotations above that women can indeed be very strongly affected by these psychological symptoms and that in many instances they may be severe enough to cause major disruption in their abilities to function on a day-to-day basis. It's interesting to note that the women's complaints are in many ways very similar to those that you might hear in connection with premenstrual tension (PMT) with the marked difference that PMT only brings about these effects for a couple of days or so during each monthly cycle.

This similarity in the complaints would once again suggest that changing hormonal levels are after all responsible for them because the PMT symptoms have been clearly identified as being caused by hormonal changes. Be that as it may, there is however a world of difference between feeling low for a couple of days because of PMT and having that same feeling for perhaps weeks on end.

Doctors in general practice are, of course, familiar with menopausal patients who present themselves with psychological symptoms. In fact, one patient symptom questionnaire suggested by a drug company for use by doctors in assessing whether a particular patient should be considered for HRT includes the following questions:

- Do you lack confidence? For example, are you unwilling to go out, or fearful of entertaining, or fear going into a supermarket?
- Are you in a depressed or anxious mood?
- Are you experiencing any of the following: lethargy/loss of energy/tiredness?
- Are you having loss of memory or concentration?

The implication of the inclusion of these queries in the questionnaire is, of course, that patients answering 'yes' to any of them are likely to need or derive benefit from HRT. Whether that is so or not still remains – as has been seen above – a debatable matter. It does however underline once again that as far as the vast majority of women are concerned, the menopause and certain symptoms are inextricably linked – and that this is also probably nowadays what most doctors accept on a practical level.

Middle age, of course, is generally marked by all sorts of difficulties, not all of them by any means connected directly to the menopause, but happening around the same time. For women in particular the late forties and early fifties are frequently watershed years when they often have to come to terms with all kinds of problems associated with that time of life and these may include:

- Children getting married or leaving home, thereby creating the so-called 'empty nest syndrome'.
- Having to accept the fact that they are aging and, whilst not yet old, they are no longer young.
- The early signs that good health is no longer something that can be taken as much for granted as it might have been in the past.
- Work may have become unfulfilling and, additionally, there may be worries about impending retirement.
- Alterations in sexual patterns, possibly leading to dissatisfaction or frustration.
- One or more bereavements in the immediate family circle, particularly that of parents or even spouse.
- And, of course, worrying about the menopause itself!

Taking the above into account, it is little wonder that menopausal women may exhibit outward signs of the difficulties they're having in coping psychologically with all the changes that are rapidly taking place around them, and that these signs also may manifest themselves in a variety of ways. Let us now look at some of these specific problems one by one and at the same time, where relevant, suggest using coping strategies that other women have reported as being helpful to them.

THE EMPTY NEST SYNDROME

The interesting thing about this is that, according to in-depth interviews with women who originally said they had been strongly affected by their last child leaving the parental home, it was found that what really mattered most to them was not so much the fact of the 'empty nest', but rather that they were having great trouble in finding a new role for themselves.

"My days were all mapped out for me until my last son got married as there were specific tasks that had to be done all the time," was one typical comment. "Now, with just my husband and myself to look after, there's just not enough to do to fill the time and I find that I'm spending many long hours just sitting around and being bored."

Another woman said: "I used to complain about being rushed off my feet because the children always wanted one thing or another. No one asks for anything now and that makes me feel utterly unwanted and useless."

Difficult though it is for women who are facing an 'empty nest' to believe at the time, this is usually a very temporary crisis and one that resolves itself as the months go by and adjustment to the new situation takes place.

"Somewhere along the way, I came to the realisation that I now had the time to do all the things I had always wanted to – and it wasn't yet too late to get started on some of them," said one woman. Another reported: "It took a while, but finally – and it was a bit of a shock initially, I can tell you – it sank home to me that it truly was a great relief to no longer be tied day after day to the needs of the children and that I was suddenly freed of their demands."

Quite commonly this pattern of eventually realising that 'as one door closes, another one opens' is the experience of many women. And, of course, women can help themselves by seizing the opportunities that lie behind the newly-opened door, such as perhaps pursuing new interests and hobbies, taking longer and more frequent holidays, joining clubs and societies, spending more time with their husbands and generally using the extra leisure they now have on hand in interesting and pleasurable ways.

EVIDENCE OF AGING

For many women, what seems to them like the sudden acceleration of the aging process is one of the more unpleasant – and dreaded – aspects of the menopause. Although, as has been mentioned earlier, the severity of some of these visible signs of aging can be reduced by HRT, even this will not eradicate them completely. In any case, it's not merely the physical signs of aging that women often have difficulty in accepting, but also that they have to in a sense revise their own opinions of themselves. This is evidenced by the following quotes:

"You can kid yourself that you're still quite young while you're under fifty – after that you just can't do it anymore."

"It's rather hard to get all that interested in the latest fashions when all you really care about is choosing clothes that will reveal the smallest possible amount of your skin because it's become so thin and wrinkled."

"I've always agreed with the idea that you're only as old as you feel. But, if your hair is thinning out and your skin has a funny kind of translucence, then it's not so easy to feel young any more."

"I know that we all get old one day – I just would have liked to postpone that day for a little while longer."

That last quotation sums up the situation in many ways: women know that their age is creeping up on them but, quite reasonably, want to postpone the outward signs as long as possible. It's all rather bad timing that quite often their looks may start to wane – or they believe that to be the case which means just about the same thing psychologically – just as they're having to cope with the menopause and all that implies as well. While it's all very well for the experts to say that we – and that includes men as well, of course – should grow older gracefully and accept each stage in life for what it is and make the most of it, the truth remains that most of us would like to hang on to relative youth a while longer. The acceptance of the fact that unfortunately there is no cure-all panacea which will stop or reverse the aging process is something we all have to come to grips with sooner or later. Obvious though it may sound, while that acceptance won't alter anything, it will make it easier to handle what's happening on a day-to-day basis.

HEALTH PROBLEMS

It is doubly unfortunate that the menopausal years are also often marked by the first signs of health not being as robust as it once was.

As with aging, this is once again part of the inexorable march of time. However, unlike aging, this is not something to be accepted quite so readily and philosophically as there usually is a great deal that can be done to make things better once again.

In fact, for many women, the menopause often brings about a re-assessment of themselves and their health. As a result of this – and the steps they take to improve matters – they may well find that eventually they are healthier than they were before. For example:

"I suppose I had let myself go while the children were growing up and it wasn't until they left home that I was able to muster the strength to go on a diet and stick to it."

"I hated reaching my fiftieth birthday, but it was also the day that I resolved that – as the phrase has it – I was going to make the best of the rest of my life. I joined a yoga class, started eating the right foods and I now feel fitter than I ever have for years."

"When I started getting the first indications that my menopause was starting, I decided there and then that although this meant I would have some unpleasant symptoms that I couldn't do anything about, I could at least make sure that I was in the best possible state of health as far as everything else was concerned. I got my doctor to give me a complete check-up and, on his advice, started a rigorous keep fit programme which has paid rich dividends. In fact, I even managed to stop smoking after going through two packs a day for nearly 30 years."

As can be seen from the above, women can manage to turn what might be a negative experience into a positive one by facing up squarely to the problems.

WORK PROBLEMS

Work can also be a great source of stress for women in their middle years as the following quotes reveal:

"I've always had a very demanding job, but generally enjoyed the challenge. Now I've reached the peak of my career and I can't help but wonder whether all the effort was really worthwhile."

"I worry intensely about the possibility of being made redundant because I know that another job will be next to impossible to find because of my age."

"My job is a very demanding one and I'm finding it more and more difficult to keep on top of it and I'm sure that my employers are noticing the fact that I'm very tired some days."

An additional related source of worry may well be concerned with the prospect of impending retirement – whether enforced or voluntary – and the reduction or loss of income that this might entail.

CHANGES IN SEXUAL PATTERNS

Not infrequently the middle years are also marked by alterations in the sexual patterns of most women. Some of these may be brought about by physical changes which are part of the menopause and this is in fact such an important area that later on a whole chapter of this book is devoted to it.

BEREAVEMENTS

Quite often a woman's menopausal years coincide with her first experience of bereavement as she suffers the loss of a parent, grandparent or other close relative. The grief which is natural at this time may just be one more factor that overloads her emotional resources. For example:

"I was going through what was probably the worst part of my menopause when my father died suddenly. His death would have been difficult to cope with at any time, but just then it was just about impossible."

"My sister was eleven years older than I and when she died after having been ill only a short time I realised how tenuous everyone's hold on life was, including my own."

"My mother's death was not unexpected as she had been very ill for many months. Yet when it happened my despair was so deep that it took several years before I began to recover from it."

WORRYING ABOUT THE MENOPAUSE

Apart from the stresses that may be brought about by events like those described above, there remains one more major source of concern – and that is worrying about the menopause itself and its effects. The extent of that worry varies considerably from woman to woman but it is shared to some extent by most:

"I remember all too clearly the years of misery my mother suffered when she had her change of life and couldn't help but think that mine might be just as bad."

"I can't bear the idea that everything is going to be thrown into turmoil by a few hormones after I thought I'd finally managed to sort out my life nicely."

"You hear such terrible stories of what other women have gone through that you can't help being a little bit scared by what is waiting for you."

"The menopause? No, I haven't worried about it at all and I must be about halfway through it by now. I just take each day as it comes."

IN CONCLUSION

Of course, the various problems outlined above aren't all experienced by all menopausal women. Nevertheless, enough of these difficulties are sufficiently more likely to occur in the middle years to ensure that they frequently are part of a pattern which can create feelings of depression during the menopause. It is these feelings – and what can be done about them – which are explored in the next chapter.

4 Depression And The Menopause

As has been seen in the previous chapter, all kinds of psychological problems form part of the menopausal years and one of the major associated symptoms is covered by the catch-all description of 'depression'. What exactly is meant by depression? It is, in fact, such a broad term that it covers all kinds of things, many of them, strictly speaking, not being depression at all.

Before going on to look at how depression – and its attendant symptoms – may occur as part of the menopause, it's worthwhile to briefly explore how widespread a complaint it is in the general population. Depression – and its stable-mate, anxiety – are among the most common illnesses and epidemiological studies have shown that within a given year about 15 per cent of the general population suffer from either of these. Even more revealing are the statistics relating to 'life-time' risk – that is the average chance of becoming a sufferer from a particular illness or disease – which put the likelihood of developing depression at between 20 and 26 per cent for women (as compared with between eight and twelve per cent for men).

So, with the odds being that roughly one in four women will within their lifetimes show symptoms of either depression or anxiety marked enough to warrant medical attention, it is hardly surprising that any sample of menopausal women will also automatically include a large number of depression sufferers. Just how large that number really is, is a subject that is still open to debate as the evidence resulting from various surveys has proven to be either inconclusive or contradictory. Nevertheless, there is plenty of anecdotal evidence to back up the claim that the rate of depressive illness is greater during the menopausal years without necessarily being able to prove just how much greater that rate is.

The situation is further confused by various factions within the medical profession disagreeing as to exactly what constitutes depression and what is anxiety. Some psychiatrists argue strongly that the two disorders should be clearly split in separate groups while others – known colloquially as 'the lumpers' – maintain that anxiety and depression are so strongly linked that they should be seen as an entity.

The argument put forward by 'the splitters' to justify the separation of depression and anxiety is that this distinction can be seen not only in the symptoms that are presented by the patients, but also in the course that the illness is likely to follow and how it will respond to treatment.

On the other hand, 'the lumpers' back up their views by citing the evidence from numerous epidemiological studies which have consistently shown that there is a substantial overlap between the two conditions and that many patients equally fulfil the criteria for a diagnosis of depression or for one of anxiety.

It is doubtful whether this argument about whether to 'lump' or 'split' depression and anxiety is likely to be resolved in the near future. In the meantime, however, on a practical basis there are several internationally recognised rating scales which doctors can use to determine whether a patient is suffering from depression or anxiety. Although these rating scales vary somewhat in the emphasis they attach to various symptoms, they coincide frequently enough and as a generality the symptoms of depression and anxiety can be compared as follows – this information being based on the *Montgomery and Asberg Depression Rating Scale*, the *Hamilton Depression Rating Scale*, and the *Hamilton Anxiety Scale*:

Symptoms seen in anxiety: Inner tension, difficulties in concentration and/or intellectual capacity, anxious mood, agitation, hypochondriasis, anxious signs and/or behaviour, gastrointestinal and/or genito-urinary disturbances, fears, psychic and somatic anxiety, as well as problems connected with the cardiovascular, respiratory and automonic systems.

Symptoms seen in depression: Sadness, inner tension, pessimistic thoughts and ideas, inability to feel emotions, reduced appetite and/or sleep, suicidal thoughts, guilt, psychic and/or somatic anxiety, agitation, loss of weight, loss of insight, difficulties in concentration, reduced sexual drive, depressed mood, as well as cardiovascular, autonomic and general somatic symptoms.

It's quite obvious from the above lists that it is indeed no easy matter to categorise a patient as falling into one group or another, as quite a few of the symptoms can be equally indicative of either depression or anxiety. Naturally enough, anxiety is frequently part of the depressive pattern while anxiety itself is recognised as one of the most frequently observed symptoms of depression.

While the medical profession may agree to continue to disagree as to whether anxiety and depression should or should not be seen as two different illnesses, the fact remains that for the majority of patients the difference matters but little. The word 'depression' is the one most commonly used by the general public to describe feeling 'mentally and emotionally low'.

Menopausal women describing their symptoms are more likely to talk of depression than about anxiety, using the term 'depression' to indicate their state of mind in general and usually mentioning anxiety only when relating it to specific worries. For example:

"I'm depressed most of the time and when I think that this is just the beginning of the menopause, I can become really anxious about it."

"All my worries just seem to pile up on top of each other and I become really depressed about it all."

"I don't know whether I'm depressed because of the menopause or whether the menopause is making me depressed."

While, as has been shown in the previous chapter, depressive symptoms are part and parcel of the menopausal process for many women, it is yet another matter whether these symptoms are severe enough to add up to actual depressive illness. And in many ways the question that poses itself is "Are the symptoms such that they require or would benefit from treatment?" rather than whether the root-cause may be anxiety or depression. Oddly enough, the treatment that may be offered may be very similar whatever the diagnosis as it has been found in recent years that many traditional forms of antidepressants are also equally effective in treating anxiety states. So it could well be that a doctor may not wish to agonise too long as to whether the patient is depressed or anxious because the treatment of choice will be the same in either instance.

What matters perhaps more as far as the average menopausal patient is concerned is what the likelihood is that she will receive a sympathetic hearing and the correct treatment when she reports her depressive symptoms to the average doctor. Sadly, it must be reported that although things are improving generally, it still remains very much a question of luck whether or not your doctor will even correctly diagnose depression. This was revealed in a paper published in 1985 in the *British Medical Journal* (Unrecognised depression in general practice) which said that about half the cases of depression – including those which were severe – were likely to remain unrecognised. And these findings apply to depression in general – not just that which happens during the menopause when doctors are all that more likely to dismiss symptoms as 'just being part of the overall pattern'.

This casual dismissal of their symptoms is, of course, deeply resented by many women in their middle years:

"When I told my doctor that there were days when I felt so low in myself that I couldn't even face going out to do the shopping, he sort of smiled and said: 'Well, we all have days when we don't feel too well'."

"My doctor is the kind of man who seems to be only interested in you when you're complaining about something straightforward, like an upset tummy or a tight chest. And it's obvious by the change in his manner that he simply switches off his mind the moment you begin to talk about how you feel inside."

"Although my doctor is a middle-aged woman and I guess must have gone through the menopause herself, she cuts me short whenever I try to raise the question of feeling down, and will quickly tell me in a rather patronising way, 'Well, you must try not to worry about things too much'."

Complaints about this lack of interest shown by some – and the word 'some' must be stressed in this context – doctors in hearing about patients' depressive symptoms came up time and time again in interviews. Yet, for many women in their middle years, the mood changes that frequently accompany the menopause – whether caused by it or not – are severe enough to warrant treatment in their own right. Of course, it also follows that doctors may miss diagnosing clinical depression or anxiety when they close their minds to what their patients are saying. This attitude, it must be assumed, is making its own contribution to the finding that about half of the cases of depression remain undiagnosed initially.

Incidentally, it is worthwhile to record briefly what the main signs – often called 'the core symptoms' – of depression are. Once again, there are several different rating scales and the following information is based upon the common factors of three of those scales: reported or observed sadness, inner tensions, loss of interest or pleasure, poor appetite, weight loss or gain – but only rarely the latter, sleep difficulties, reduced concentration, loss of energy or fatigue, feelings of self-reproach and/or guilt, recurrent suicidal thoughts or thoughts of death.

Although at first glance this list appears quite similar to that which was used to distinguish depression from anxiety, there is one important difference because the number of 'core symptoms' is used by many doctors to determine whether depression is present and whether it requires treatment. And this diagnostic system works out as follows: the criteria for a diagnosis of major depression are met when at least five core symptoms, one of which must be sadness, have been observed.

Although the 'five symptoms' test is one that is used quite frequently by doctors, it is felt by some that this can be too stringent and they instead prefer to follow a variation of it which works out as follows:

Depression can be diagnosed if the following three conditions are met:

1) Anxiety and/or depression complaints are present.
2) The symptoms have been present for longer than two weeks.
3) At least three core symptoms have been identified in which case the diagnosis is probably depression, but not necessarily demanding treatment; if four or more core symptoms are found, then the diagnosis is that of depression requiring treatment.

Naturally enough, any such test must be applied with common sense and due allowance made for the relative severity of the core symptoms. Nevertheless, this yardstick used by many family doctors can also be used by individuals as a simple way of finding out whether they are 'feeling depressed' or are actually suffering from depression and therefore should seek medical help. While such self-diagnosis can be helpful, it must be stressed that anyone suffering the symptoms of depression or anxiety – whether or not these are 'core symptoms' – for any length of time should seek medical advice, if only for the reassurance that this might bring.

Reassurance is often one of the main benefits that a doctor can offer a menopausal patient in the first instance. Commented one family doctor: "Most of the patients we see present symptoms that might be indicative of depression, but are much more likely to be mild anxiety. And one way to approach these situations is to provide reassurance while waiting to see whether a treatable illness does in fact emerge. Generally, it is best to provide this reassurance over several visits so that the patient can be observed over a period of time and any improvement or worsening of the symptoms duly noted. In many instances, no illness will follow and what you might call 'therapeutic listening' will have been enough to help allay the patient's fears in the meantime. And, should symptoms indicating a more severe disturbance come to light later, this initial assessment period ensures that it will be recognised as early as possible."

That reassurance that their symptoms are not necessarily indicative of serious problems can be both needed and sought by menopausal women as indicated by the following quotes:

"I tell myself that feeling low is a normal part of the menopause and I must expect this to happen now and again. However, I just wish that my doctor would be willing to spend a little more time with me and make sure that there's nothing else wrong with me."

"It's a vicious circle – I get the blues, then I start to worry about feeling a bit depressed, and end up being depressed about being depressed. I'd really like someone who knows what he's talking about to tell me that what I'm undergoing is normal and that I'm not going out of my mind."

"A friend of mine did become severely depressed when she had her menopause, so severely that she was on high dosage antidepressants for many months. I'm now having occasional anxiety attacks, and I know that these are probably not very meaningful. Yet it would help me such a lot if I could be told that there is nothing to worry about in my case."

Other in-depth interviews with menopausal women have also frequently highlighted their belief that a sympathetic hearing coupled with reassurance based on knowledge would go a long way towards making it easier for them to cope with the symptoms of anxiety or depression. "It's not that we're becoming psychological hypochondriacs because we're menopausal," said one woman, "but rather that like anyone else having unpleasant symptoms it helps to know for sure that is all they are and that they don't mean that something even worse is waiting in the wings."

There is, of course, a big difference between being reassured – by being told after the necessary examination and assessment that there is nothing to worry about – and having your symptoms airily dismissed with the statement 'you worry too much'.

It is true, of course, that most women worry about their feelings during the menopause. It is quite another thing altogether to suggest that they worry too much. It's perfectly natural and reasonable for a woman who is experiencing some psychological symptoms to worry about them even though she is perfectly aware that the chances are that these symptoms are minor and will probably disappear of their own accord with the passage of time. That's where a sympathetic hearing by a doctor who is seen to be interested and concerned can work wonders as fears are allayed by reassurance which also automatically reduces the patient's anxiety.

However, while reassurance may be enough in many instances, there are, of course, many cases where the symptoms of depression or anxiety are sufficiently severe to warrant treatment. Which form that treatment should take will vary considerably from case to case, but until recently the *benzodiazepines* were likely to be the first line of defence against anxiety symptoms. First introduced in 1960, the benzodiazepines – of which *diazepam* and *lorazepam* were probably the most widely prescribed – often brought rapid relief to the patient by eliminating symptoms while producing few or no side-effects. In later years, however, the medical profession became increasingly concerned by the number of patients receiving the medication as well as the length of time they remained on it. Since then, the *Committee on Safety of Medicines* has recommended that benzodiazepines – while indicated for the short-term relief of severe or disabling anxiety – were inappropriate and unsuitable for the treatment of short-term 'mild' anxiety.

However, it remains to be said that this recommendation is by no means fully observed by many family doctors and that the benzodiazepines, despite their shortcomings, continue to be frequently prescribed for the relief of comparatively mild anxiety.

As has been mentioned earlier, it has been found that *antidepressants* are often more effective in the treatment of anxiety than some of the drugs intended specifically for that purpose, such as the benzodiazepines, and there usually is a smaller risk of eventual dependence. There are, however, also many problems associated with the use of antidepressants in anxiety and these include the fact that they can be comparatively slow in producing their effect and this can mean that some patients may not persevere long enough with them to gain any benefit. Another problem is that some antidepressants can produce as side-effects some of the very symptoms that patients worry about most, such as irritability, insomnia and apprehension.

Another group of drugs that has been used to treat both anxiety and depression are the *MAOIs* – the initials stand for *monoamine oxidase inhibitors* – and these have been found particularly efficient in controlling panic attacks. However, great caution needs to be exercised with these as they can interact dangerously with certain foods as well as other drugs and for that reason their use is usually avoided where safer preparations are available.

The above, of course, is only a very small sample of the various drugs available to reduce anxiety or depression problems and doctors today can choose from a much wider variety of treatments than ever before. This means that any symptoms of anxiety or depression – providing these are severe enough to warrant treatment in the first instance – that you may develop during the menopause are all that much more likely to be brought swiftly under control. Perhaps the single most useful piece of advice that can be given to someone who is having difficulties with either undue anxiety or possible depression is: *Don't suffer in silence, go and see your doctor and, should you not get the help you think you need during your first visit, go back again if the symptoms persist.*

5 Sexuality And The Menopause

There are all sorts of reasons why a woman's interest in sex may reduce in the middle years. And – as with many of the physical and psychological symptoms described earlier – some of these reasons can be clearly attributed to the menopause while it is more likely that others are just part of the process of growing older.

That increasing age usually brings with it a decrease in the frequency of both intercourse and orgasm has been known ever since *Kinsey* published the results of the first major study of human sexuality in the United States. Although this was many decades ago, more recent surveys continue to reveal identical patterns.

Kinsey's findings, although advanced for their time, could be said with hindsight to be somewhat simplistic in that he used data relating solely to the frequency of intercourse and orgasm to draw conclusions about the decrease in sexual interest for both men and women. There is a problem, however, with using frequency of intercourse as the sole yardstick because it only measures the number of times that a couple's sexual drives coincide and, as such, only provides reliable evidence about the couple seen as an entity and not about the two individual persons involved.

There is now a great amount of evidence to support the general notion that, yes, frequency of intercourse diminishes with age, but that this is mainly due to men becoming sexually less active and does not necessarily represent a parallel decline of interest as far as women are concerned. And, according to a recent survey of men and women in Oxford (Study of symptoms in middle life with special reference to the menopause, G T Bungay et al, published in the *British Medical Journal*) men's sexual interest can begin to wane from as early as the late forties onwards, while women's sexual interest tends to continue at much the same levels as previously even when they reach their fifties or older.

Not only has it been observed that there often is no decline in the sex drive of women in their middle years, the most comprehensive study of female sexuality of all – *The Hite Report* by Shere Hite – concludes that for many women sexual desire may often actually increase as they become older.

So the picture that emerges is not necessarily one of older women becoming less interested in sex because of the menopause, but rather one of men's reduced libido creating a reduction in the rate of intercourse. Anecdotal support for this view is to be found in women's own accounts:

"I can't say that my menopause really affected my sex life at all as that had just about gone by the board some years earlier, more or less when my husband reached the age of fifty – perhaps he had his menopause then!"

"It's not that I have changed, but rather that my husband has. I'm just as interested in making love as I was before my menopause began; he, however, seems to think that my change of life also means the end of sex."

"No, we don't have sex very often, but this is hardly news as it has been that way for years. This doesn't mean that we don't enjoy making love when we do – it's just that it doesn't happen very often. I suppose I personally would prefer it if it happened more often, but then it takes two to agree to tango, doesn't it?"

While surveys tend broadly to agree that in general women's interest in sex doesn't necessarily diminish and may quite often even increase in the middle years, there is also substantial evidence to show that some women at least do see the menopause as a time when sexual activity naturally begins to lessen, as exemplified by the following quotes:

"Although I'm not one of those people who believe that sex should only be indulged in for the purpose of procreation, I do think that I looked upon lovemaking somewhat differently once I could no longer have babies."

"For years I had thought that our sex life could be somewhat better, but never really did anything much about it. I suppose that I used the menopause as a handy excuse for leaving things as they were because, after all, it was a bit late in the day then, wasn't it?"

"Sex is great for the young, but surely it does become less important as you get older."

"I've never really quite understood all this emphasis on sex and admit that I had always seen one of the benefits of the menopause as being a kind of natural end to that chapter."

Of course, what these quotations illustrate, is that in many instances a woman's reaction to the menopause – whether concerned with sexuality or other matters – is very likely to be influenced by opinions formed and held for years before. If sex wasn't very important to a woman when she was young, then the chances are that it will matter even less as she becomes older. On the other hand, a woman whose sex drive has always been robust may find that the menopause has but little effect upon it.

It is naturally always somewhat dangerous to quote statistical evidence in connection with what is after all a very individual activity, as comparisons with 'norms' can be distinctly unhelpful. Having said that, statistics do help paint the broader picture and many women are extremely interested in seeing how their experiences may match those of others.

As explained above, the frequency of intercourse by itself can be a poor measure of sexual interest, as sex in that form is dependent upon the availability of a suitable and willing partner. More revealing in many ways is frequency of sexual activity, as this term includes both intercourse and self-stimulation. And the following figures – derived from a study in America by the *Consumers Union* of some 1,800 women, three quarters of whom were married – does show the incidence of activity in different age groups:

Women aged over 50 years. 88 per cent were found to be sexually active with 73 per cent reporting sexual activity as taking place at least once a week; 47 per cent also reported self-stimulation.

Women aged over 60 years. The number of sexually active women had dropped to 63 per cent with an identical number being sexually active at least once a week; there was also a substantial decrease – down to 37 per cent – in the numbers of those reporting self-stimulation.

Women aged over 70 years. Exactly half – 50 per cent – of women still remained sexually active and were so at least once a week. Interestingly, the percentage of those who reported self-stimulation was 37 per cent, the same as for those aged over 60 years.

Surprising though these figures may be to some, they are only part of the evidence that sexual activity doesn't reduce as much with thc passing years as younger people might be led into supposing. What's more, there is a firm belief amongst researchers that the statistics tell just a small part of the story because they are only concerned with sexual activity that actually happens and don't necessarily reflect how much such activity older women might choose if the opportunities were available.

"Many older women live alone, having been either divorced or widowed", remarked one researcher, "and therefore may well have difficulties in finding suitable partners. Additionally, ill health may also play a role in reducing sexual interest.

"And even for those women whose husbands or partners are still alive and living with them, there may still be problems which affect sexual activity, such as illness of the partner or apathy from his side. And, of course, erection problems become more common as men get older and this may make its own negative contribution to the situation. So, quite often, it's not so much a question of the woman no longer wishing to have sex, but that circumstances make it either so unfulfilling or frustrating that she gradually loses interest."

While some of the above paints a somewhat dismal view of the chances of the woman in her middle years having a satisfactory sex life, there is another, much more positive, side with many women finding that the menopause actually has a beneficial effect. One of the factors frequently mentioned by women who found this to be the case is that they were freed of the fear of an unwanted pregnancy. Others said that the menopause brought home to them the fact that the years were slipping by and that this realisation led them to resolve that they would make the most of the remaining ones. Quite frequently women who were receiving HRT reported that this had also rejuvenated them sexually.

But, whatever the reasons may be, the menopause can be a tonic to revive flagging sexual interest as the following quotations testify:

"When I was younger, it seemed as though my periods were always falling on just the wrong days, the ones when my husband was feeling romantic. And we hardly ever managed to get our sexual calendars to synchronise. Talk about star-crossed lovers, indeed! Now, with that problem nicely out of the way, sex is not only more frequent but better as well."

"I never did like all the paraphernalia involved in birth control and it has always been a real put-off for me. How can sex be enjoyable if you have to fiddle around with various gadgets first? Thankfully, I'm now safely past the menopause and my no longer having to worry about possibly becoming pregnant means that sex can be spontaneous . . . and, in my case at least, that has meant more frequent as well."

"It may sound strange, but I actually discovered 'sex lib', if not 'women's lib', when my menopause started. Knowing that this was an important stage in my life, I read as much about it as possible and along the way found a whole wealth of information about female sexuality. And that is how I also learned why until then sex had been less than satisfactory for me because rather naively I had been expecting vaginal rather than clitoral stimulation to give me orgasms. Suddenly, a whole new world of sexual enjoyment had opened up to me . . ."

Stories like the ones above crop up time and time again when women are asked about their sex lives during and after the menopause. Remarked one psychologist: "It's as though being menopausal gives some women a kind of new freedom. Until then, they had seen their roles in life very narrowly, that of being a good wife and a good mother. There is another facet that I have encountered frequently and that is that women are initially shocked – and that's not too strong a word – by the menopause when its first signs appear and somewhat later, perhaps as part of their adjustment to this shock, decide that they will now become their 'own person'. This new spirit of independence can cause them to alter their views drastically about all sorts of things and, naturally enough, that includes sex as well."

The rekindling of sexual desire in women in their middle years can often bring its own problems as they are often married to men whose own sexual drives are flagging. The situation may be further worsened by the husband having perhaps sought sexual reassurance by getting involved with another – usually younger – woman and showing even less physical interest in his wife.

The combination of a philandering husband and a wife who is eager to enjoy sex more fully is an explosive one and probably accounts partly for the high separation and divorce rates for couples in their late forties and early fifties.

The choices faced by the middle-aged woman who is saddled with a husband or partner who doesn't share her enthusiasm for rediscovering sexual pleasures are few. One option is to find herself a lover, something that is not always done all that easily and may also not be acceptable to her own personal moral code. Another possibility is to break off her current relationship and set off alone in her brave new world in the hope of finding a new partner and starting life all over again. Then there is another choice - and that is to contain and suppress her sexual appetites.

As can be imagined, each of these options is likely to bring its own problems and so all too often what follows is that the woman 'hangs on' in the vague hope that sooner or later 'things will get better'. What happens usually in those cases is not so much a question of things getting better, but that they settle down, as the woman – with varying degrees of resentment and resignation – begins to accept with reluctance that after all 'there are more important things in life than sex'.

So far this chapter has been concerned with sexual desire and activity as purely physical manifestations which can be quantified and measured by data about such things as the frequency of intercourse and how often orgasms occur. Yet, there's a good deal more to sexuality than that and this was made particularly apparent in how menopausal women described their needs:

"Although I still want physical closeness and satisfaction, that has really become the lesser part of my needs. What I really care about is to feel that my husband still loves me. If there's less sex nowadays, so be it, just as long as there's enough affectionate touching, kissing and cuddling."

"What I resent most about the menopause is how my partner just assumed that it meant the end of sex for us. The thing that really grates on me is that he decided this all by himself without even bothering discussing it first with me and finding out how I might feel about it. It seemed as though a label had been stuck on my forehead saying: 'This woman is menopausal – Do not touch!'."

"I'd just like to be told now and then that I look good or that my hair is nice or that my dress is becoming. My husband never was the greatest at handing out compliments, but now he never comments one way or another."

"I can accept the lack of physical contact – note that I say 'accept it', not like it – but what's driving me around the bend is that it seems that I've become a non-person as far as my partner is concerned. As well as a warm and satisfying physical relationship, we also used to have what I can only call a mental togetherness in that we would talk for hours on end about everything under the sun. That, too, has gone out of the window . . ."

"You know, when most women talk about a sexual relationship they're really not all that concerned about physical contact. What they're on about is both giving and receiving affection."

So it seems that resentment – mixed with regret – is quite frequently brought about by the menopause when some women find themselves pitched against their will into a new role, one which they both dislike and reject. This rejection often centres not so much around sexual activity as such, but is more likely to be focused upon the image – both self-perceived and as reflected by the actions and views of others – of their desirability.

The message that desirability is a 'good thing' has been drummed time and time again over the years into the heads of all of us, men and women alike. Advertisers promote their products by showing us young, lithe bodies and warn us of the perils of wrinkled skin or gaining an extra pound of fat. While the purpose of all this may be to shift more goods off the shelves, the underlying message remains that if you don't match the stereotypes of physical beauty that constantly surround you, then you're not likely to be a satisfactory person, let alone a sexually desirable one.

If it can be difficult at times for a comparatively young woman even to begin to match these media-imposed criteria of desirability, then how much more so it is for a woman of mature years. "I never thought of myself as particularly attractive to men", said one woman, "but at least I had age on my side. Now even that is gone."

It can, of course, be argued that women shouldn't perhaps try so hard to appear younger as they go into their fifties and sixties. But the fact remains – no matter what extreme supporters of the Women's Liberation movement may proclaim – that most women, whatever their ages, want to look good and feel good. And for most to look good is to feel good – or at least not feel bad.

'Looking good' all too often means looking young and it is unreasonable to expect that equation to change for the time being. Idealists who advance the notion that women should be valued for 'what they are' and not for 'what they look like' may find that there is much agreement for this in principle. In practice, however, most women will still continue to put personal appearance high on their lists of priorities.

Whether or not the media and its stereotyped images is mainly to blame or not for this is perhaps only of academic interest and what really matters is how women themselves react to the visible signs of aging:

"What is it that the song says? 'Nobody wants you when you're old and grey', isn't it? Well, that sums up my experience, too."

"Sure I care whether I get wrinkles or I wouldn't have spent a fortune on oil-of-you-know-what over the years."

"It's okay for a man if his face gets a few lines, it just makes it more interesting. Wrinkles on a woman – why she is suddenly middle-aged!"

"In an ideal world, women – and men too for that matter – should be allowed to grow older gracefully without any pressures on them to remain perpetually young. But then it's hardly an ideal world, is it?"

The underlying theme of these quotations is that many women are well aware of the various pressures that insist they should continue looking young and desirable even though in many cases the pressures are resented strongly by them intellectually. Despite that resentment, most women will give in to these demands of the outside world to a greater or lesser degree for all sorts of reasons – often perhaps because they believe that this is what they have to do to hang on to a man or a job.

Like it or not, in today's world sexuality and good looks are connected and the most intelligent, charming and sensual woman will still at the very least be partially judged by others on her appearance. We're all familiar with how the very opposite type – the woman who has but little to recommend her but her looks – will seldom lack admirers. This is perhaps not as it should be, but the way it is.

While statistics abound about all sorts of aspects of the menopause, it remains, of course, quite impossible to predict how an individual woman may choose to handle her change of life years. That is a very personal decision and one that only she can make for herself. What may be right for one woman might not be so for another. What's more, in the sexual context we're talking about three highly variable elements: the woman's own philosophy and outlook on life in general; how the menopause affects her physically and emotionally; and – perhaps the most important variable of them all – what her own natural sexuality and desires are, not just during the menopausal years, but also before that and afterwards.

There is, however, one factor that is so common to all individual experiences that it is worthy of mention. Women, generally much more so than men (no matter what the men themselves might choose to believe), are essentially pragmatic creatures. This pragmatism is reflected by another philosophical thread which ran through much of what those interviewed by researchers had to say about sex and the menopause – yes, there often were problems; and, also yes, their situations often weren't much to their liking; and, most emphatically yes, they made the best of what was possible.

Fortunately – setting aside for a moment the potential benefits of HRT – there are many practical things that women can do to ensure that they keep looking good and feeling good during the middle years and these are covered in detail in a later chapter.

Before going on to that, however, there is one sexual aspect of the menopause that deliberately has not been mentioned so far: how the altering hormonal levels often bring with them specific physical changes that can affect a woman's enjoyment – and therefore her desire – for sex. That is what the next chapter is all about.

6 Genito-Urinary Changes During The Menopause

Apart from the changes in sexual outlook and desire which may take place during the menopause and which have been explored in the previous chapter, the middle years are also a time when specific physical changes occur and some of these can have a marked effect upon sexuality.

As has been described previously, the menopause is a time when hormone levels ebb and flow and gradually reduce over a period of time. The supply to the body of one of these hormones in particular – oestrogen, the main source of which are the ovaries, although a small amount of it is also produced by other parts of the body – eventually becomes just about non-existent.

Normally, much of the oestrogen produced by a woman before the menopause is taken up by the vagina, uterus and cervix and it follows that as the hormone supply dwindles these are the organs where the effects of the deficiency are most marked. Essentially what happens is that the lack of oestrogen causes the surface tissues – or lining – to atrophy slowly. The direct consequences of this can include:

- A shortening of the vagina; the blood supply to it may be reduced and as a result its skin surface will become weaker and thinner.
- The falling oestrogen level also affects vaginal acidity and brings about a reduction in the secretions of the mucus glands. This creates dryness which in turn may cause intercourse to become uncomfortable or even painful as well as leading to a greater risk of bleeding and infection in the vagina.

- The uterus and cervix may shrink and the cervical canal become shorter.

As might be expected, these changes – especially vaginal dryness – can profoundly influence the extent to which a woman can find sex enjoyable and painful intercourse – known as '*dyspareunia*' – quite commonly results.

This, in turn, will affect the extent to which she may welcome sexual activity. That vaginal dryness adversely affects most menopausal and postmenopausal women is borne out by the results of a study conducted by the *Consumers Union* in America (the same source quoted on sexual frequency in the previous chapter) who asked 1,844 women: 'Do you find that you produce sufficient natural lubrication to make intercourse comfortable?' Only 48 per cent of women in their fifties said, yes, there was enough natural lubrication; the rate of 'yes' answers dropped to 35 per cent for women in their sixties; and a further drop to just 23 per cent was recorded for those in their seventies.

It's quite clear from the above that vaginal dryness is a widespread problem, affecting as it does roughly one woman in three over the age of fifty. The statistics, of course, only reveal its incidence and not how much of a problem it can really be for individuals. For that, one has to rely upon what women themselves had to say about it:

"How can you be expected to enjoy sex if it feels as though sandpaper is being rubbed against you?"

"My husband and I used to have a very satisfactory sex life. Then in the later part of the menopause, my vagina became drier and drier. In fact it was so dry that he found it almost impossible to achieve penetration and when he did I quite frequently had to ask him to stop."

"After years of worrying about possible pregnancy, I was looking forward to when that wouldn't interfere any more with my enjoyment of sex. But far from being enjoyable, I now find that sex is so acutely painful that I've lost all interest."

"The very idea of having sex has now become repellent to me as I find it so uncomfortable that I use every possible excuse to avoid it. Yes, vaginal dryness has made me become one of those women who always plead a headache as a stock excuse."

Although vaginal dryness – the medical term for which is '*atrophic vaginitis*' – can present severe difficulties, its effects can usually be brought under control fairly easily.

Essentially, there are two main approaches to solving the problem. One of these is to use *locally applied oestrogen therapy* and details of this will be found in a later chapter which covers all aspects of HRT. The other, simpler solution is to use an *artificial lubricant* to replace or supplement the vagina's natural lubrication. The lubricant is either applied gently over the man's erect penis or carefully introduced into the vagina before penetration.

In the past, petroleum jelly had often been used for this purpose, but as it is not water soluble it can therefore adhere to the vaginal walls and possibly hide symptoms of infection. Additionally, petroleum jelly has been found on occasions to irritate vaginal tissues if these are particularly sensitive. Another everyday product that is sometimes used is baby oil, but that of course is also oil-based and hence not water soluble. A further problem with oil-based lubricants is that they can damage rubber condoms, an important factor if these are used for birth control. In fact, tests have shown that the strength of a condom can be reduced by up to 95 per cent within 15 minutes of contact with certain oil-based products.

Although it is not the purpose of this book to promote any particular manufacturer's products, there is one lubricating agent – *K-Y* Jelly* – whose use is so widespread and name so well-known that it would be rather senseless to describe it other than by its trade name. The big advantage that this jelly offers over most other products is that it is water soluble which means that it will naturally wash out of the vagina and is unlikely to irritate even the most sensitive of tissues. Additionally, if used with a condom, it has been shown that the extra lubrication reduces the likelihood of the condom tearing.

You don't have to have a doctor's prescription to buy this jelly which is usually supplied in a tube. Recently, however, it has also been launched on the market in the form of a smooth, solid pessary which can be simply inserted in the vagina before intercourse where it will quickly soften to a gel. Obviously, the use of a pessary can be more discreet than that of a jelly and, say the makers, 'your partner need never know a lubricant is being used'.

A word of caution, however: although vaginal dryness during and after the menopause is almost certainly a symptomatic by-product of declining or failing oestrogen, there is always a possibility that the lack of natural lubrication may be due to other causes. Although it is naturally very tempting to put the dryness down as a normal menopausal problem and simply overcome this by using one or other artificial lubricant, this is not the recommended thing to do. If you experience vaginal dryness to any extent, you should discuss this with your doctor so that any other medical problem can be ruled out.

Finally, there is one aspect of vaginal dryness that, perhaps, is so obvious that it shouldn't need stating, but stated it will be nevertheless: foreplay before intercourse helps the woman produce her natural lubrication and it may well be that extending the length of foreplay may be enough to produce sufficient lubrication when the supply of this might otherwise be failing. What's more, it has also been found that an active sex life can help keep the sexual organs in good condition.

The message from the above is clear: vaginal dryness can be easily overcome and should not be allowed to become an obstruction to the smooth continuation of lovemaking into and after the menopausal years.

CYSTITIS

There is a fair amount of difference of opinion within the medical profession about the extent to which menopausal women may suffer from cystitis. Cystitis is inflammation of the bladder resulting in painful urination, the pain usually being felt as a burning or scalding sensation either during or immediately after urinating.

The argument resolves not so much around the question of whether the symptoms of painful urination are more common during the menopause – on this part, all authorities seem to agree that the answer is yes – but rather upon whether the cause of this is indeed cystitis.

On the one hand, for example, there is the evidence offered by cystitis specialist Ann Kilmartin, who states: "The cystitis . . . can be both bacterial or non-bacterial. Both sorts are due to aging skin." And, she adds, "Over the years in my work with women who suffer from cystitis, about one third of them start cystitis in the menopause or following a hysterectomy."

Yet, Dr Robert C D Wilson, who is currently Physician in Charge of the PMS Clinic at *Marie Stopes Clinic* in London, warns that 'symptoms of painful urination accompanied by frequency are often wrongly attributed to cystitis'. In his experience the most common cause of the cystitis-like symptoms is instead inflammation of the vagina (known as *vaginitis*) rather than of the bladder.

It is important that the root-cause of whatever is giving rise to the symptoms be correctly diagnosed as the treatment is likely to be quite different. If examination fails to reveal the presence of bacteria in either the urine or the vagina then vaginitis will be the diagnosis and the treatment offered is likely to take the form of a *topical oestrogen* – 'topical' meaning that it is administered locally as opposed to 'systemic'. Topical oestrogens are usually supplied in a cream form together with a calibrated applicator although some are also available as pessaries.

The treatment for cystitis is, however, quite different as it may even respond to the frequently recommended home-remedy of increasing one's intake of water or fruit drinks as well as taking a level teaspoonful of bicarbonate of soda dissolved in water three times a day. But even such a simple treatment should be approached with some caution as bicarbonate of soda should not be taken at the same time as other drugs as it may impair their absorption.

So, the sensible thing to do is not to try to identify for yourself whether your urinary symptoms are due to one cause or another, but to consult your doctor. A word of practical advice, when you keep your appointment, take with you a specimen of your urine as this will help speed matters along.

VAGINAL THRUSH

Thrush is an illness which is caused by a tiny yeast-like fungus called *Candida albicans* which although generally present in the body doesn't normally cause any problems as it is kept at a safe level by the body's own bacterial defence mechanisms. Under certain circumstances, however, the natural balance that keeps the yeast in check becomes upset and it breeds to levels which are too high and you get thrush, which can manifest itself as one or more of the following symptoms:

- An itching feeling around the outside of the vagina (known as *vulval pruritus*).
- Delicate tissues in and around the vagina may become swollen giving rise to soreness.
- Discomfort or pain on urination as the salty urine stings the sore tissues.
- A much heavier and thicker vaginal discharge as compared with the normal light discharge most healthy women have. The discharge linked to thrush has been described as 'white, curdy and looking somewhat like cottage cheese'.

The reasons why thrush may appear are many, but one of these is that it may appear if your general state of health isn't very good and that your body's defences against illness have become weakened. This means, of course, that it is more difficult for you to fight off all kinds of minor infections, including thrush. Some menopausal women, particularly if their symptoms are severe and they haven't received the right help for them, may find that their general state of health has indeed suffered, making them more likely to develop thrush.

Women who are taking the contraceptive pill are also more likely to develop thrush as the oestrogen in the pill increases sugar levels in the body which in turn aid the yeast to grow.

Treatment for thrush is usually a fairly straightforward matter for your doctor once the initial diagnosis has been made. First of all, there are topical treatments – either in cream or pessary form – which work extremely well, but there are also newer forms of therapy which can be taken by mouth when one day's treatment is usually sufficient.

While vaginal thrush can be extremely unpleasant and embarrassing, it is unlikely to develop into anything more serious. However, it is an ailment about which there are many misconceptions and it's just as well to clear these up:

- Vaginal thrush is not a venereal disease and isn't usually caught from another person. However, it can be transmitted by sexual contact. Additionally, as intercourse may cause damage to the vaginal tissues, this can precipitate an attack of thrush.
- Thrush can also affect other parts of the body which are warm and moist, such as the mouth and folds in the skin under the breasts and around the groin.
- It's not just women who can have thrush as it can also affect men and even babies. Men will frequently have no symptoms but if they do it is likely to take the form of an inflammation of the penis.

Although the correct treatment will usually bring the condition quickly under control, there are several things you can do afterwards to stop thrush from coming back:

- Wear cotton underwear and choose stockings rather than tights. If you do wear tights, go for those which have an open or cotton gusset.
- Loose-fitting skirts and baggy trousers are a better bet because of the extra ventilation they provide as compared with tighter garments.
- Try to reduce your intake of sugar.
- Use sanitary towels rather than tampons and never use perfumed tampons.
- When washing yourself, do so gently and never harshly. Avoid using water that is very hot.
- When towelling yourself dry, don't rub too hard; pat off the

dampness instead. Changing towels and flannels frequently is also a good idea.

- Avoid perfumed preparations such as many soaps, bubble baths, vaginal deodorants, douches and antiseptics.
- Avoid inadvertently carrying infection to the vagina from the bowel by wiping from the front to the back after a bowel movement.

URINARY INCONTINENCE

An additional problem that may be faced by women in their menopause is that of urinary incontinence – that is the involuntary loss of urine – which is more likely to manifest itself at that time.

There are essentially two reasons why this should happen. First of all, the drop in oestrogen levels that can cause the shrinking of vagina, uterus and cervix may also similarly affect the bladder, which stores urine, as well as the urethra, the flexible conduit which leads from the bladder to the outside of the body. One or more of these changes may give rise to incontinence.

Secondly, the hormonal changes can also weaken the pelvic floor muscles. These muscles lie across the human pelvis and act to support in the first instance the pelvic organs, that is the bladder, rectum and uterus, but also support the abdominal contents when you're standing up. The urethra in its journey down from the bladder passes through these muscles and the external sphincter – which is the valve which opens to release urine into the urethra – virtually forms part of them. So it follows that the condition of the pelvic floor muscles can greatly influence how well the sphincter does its job of controlling the flow of urine.

While there are many different sorts of incontinence, the two types most commonly associated with the menopause are:

URGE INCONTINENCE. This can be best described as a condition that causes a sudden desire to rush urgently to the toilet to get there in time. Other symptoms may include a need to pass urine frequently – say, more than about six times a day and perhaps once at night –

and an occasional wetted bed.

STRESS INCONTINENCE. The 'stress' referred to here is actual physical stress, not mental or emotional stress as some might think. This type of incontinence is characterised by the occasional and involuntary loss of urine when you cough, sneeze or laugh. Leakages may also happen while you're making a fairly strenuous physical effort such as jogging or bending over to lift a heavy object.

Once again it must be pointed out that while occasional urinary incontinence is quite frequently part of the menopausal pattern and generally is not particularly medically significant, it should always be brought to the attention of your doctor. There are several good reasons why you should do this:

1) Incontinence, even in a mild degree, can be an extremely unpleasant disorder which can easily make your life miserable unless brought swiftly under control.
2) As with any other problem, the sooner treatment is started, the sooner a cure is likely to follow.
3) Although urinary incontinence experienced during the menopause is almost certainly due to the effects of changing hormone levels, it is, of course, possible that there may be other reasons for it. These other possibilities can only be excluded by a thorough medical examination.

Women, not unnaturally, are particularly reticent about incontinence and the evidence is that too many prefer to suffer the symptoms in silence rather than seek help from their doctor. This situation is not helped by the fact that many women who had children will have had some experience of incontinence after childbirth and that this may have disappeared of its own accord with the passage of time. So, when faced with what appears to be a similar problem later in their lives, they will tell themselves that this too is a temporary difficulty and all they have to do is wait for it to go away. Unfortunately, the course that incontinence may follow during the menopause is by no means always the same as that which it may take if it has been precipitated by childbirth. It is therefore essential that you should see your doctor if you have any leakage of urine to seek his advice.

The treatment of incontinence will, of course, be dependent upon its cause, and quite often a series of exercises may be all that's needed to restore full control.

If the diagnosis is one of urge incontinence, that's the one that causes you to rush frequently and suddenly to the toilet, then the answer might lie in learning one of several techniques which have the common aim of enabling you to delay voluntarily going to the toilet by 're-training' your bladder. Perhaps the best known and most popular of these techniques is the so-called '*pelvic floor muscles squeeze*' – which can also be used to control the symptoms of stress incontinence.

To use the squeeze, you need first of all to locate and identify the sphincter muscle that controls the release of urine. The easiest way to do this is by going to the toilet when you have a moderately full bladder and start to urinate. Once the stream has started, try to stop its flow. If your pelvic floor muscles are quite weak, you may find it impossible to stop the flow completely, but you will be using the right muscles if it slows even slightly. After stopping – or slowing – the flow, relax and empty your bladder fully. After practising this a few times on different occasions, you will find it easy to stop and start the flow at will by producing the 'squeeze'.

Having identified the 'squeeze', the next step is to strengthen it by a regular programme of exercises. There are several possible recommended routines for these exercises – which incidentally should be done when you don't feel a particular need to urinate – which can otherwise be done at any time.

Exercise routine 1. Perform the squeeze and hold it for three seconds, then let go for one second. This 'three and one' sequence should be repeated six times and the whole routine three times a day for the first week or so. After that gradually increase the number of sequences to 12 at a time, the whole routine being repeated three times daily.

Exercise routine 2. Known as the 'one and one' routine, this requires you to 'squeeze' tightly for one second only before relaxing also for only one second, after which you squeeze and relax alternatively for up to 20 times. This routine should be performed three times daily and as you become more adept at it, you should try to speed up the rate of contractions.

Exercise routine 3. This is perhaps the most difficult of the lot and consists of squeezing for ten seconds before relaxing for five seconds and then going on to the next squeeze. This should be repeated five times and the whole routine performed three times daily. Be warned, however, it may be difficult at first to hold the squeeze for the whole ten seconds and you may have to practise quite a lot before you reach that stage.

Which particular set of routines you choose is up to you and they all have equally good records in achieving the desired aim of improving sphincter control.

While this improved control may be enough to restore continence, the squeeze technique may also be used in other ways to deal specifically with either urge or stress incontinence.

THE 'SQUEEZE' FOR URGE INCONTINENCE

When you feel the need to urinate:

- Sit down and keep still as it's easier to control the urge while not moving.
- Do several quick squeezes in succession without relaxing fully between them.
- Relax generally, perhaps taking a few deep breaths.
- Use your mind to suppress the urgency feeling and continue doing so until it has either gone or virtually done so.
- Once the urge has subsided, go to the toilet in an unhurried way (it may help to continue to exert squeezes as you walk) and once you get there, release the urine in a controlled way.

THE 'SQUEEZE' FOR STRESS INCONTINENCE

As explained earlier, stress incontinence occurs as the result of a specific action, such as sneezing, laughing, coughing and so on, and these actions which cause leakages to occur can be considered as 'trigger points'. Here's how you use the squeeze to establish bladder control whenever you're doing something that is a trigger point for you:

- As soon as you become aware that you're doing something – or even better yet, about to do something that is a trigger point – squeeze immediately just before and during the time of the activity.
- If the activity is a protracted one, such as jogging, you obviously won't be able to keep on squeezing all the time. The answer in this instance is to practise rhythmic squeezing, that is, squeeze a couple of times or so, then relax for half a minute or so, then squeeze twice again.

Obviously, although you'll be using the squeeze at specific times to provide bladder control when it's particularly likely to be needed, you should also continue with the exercise routines outlined at the beginning of this section so that the muscles you've worked so hard to re-train are not allowed to lose their new strength.

7 Osteoporosis And The Menopause

Although quite naturally enough women will in the first instance be primarily concerned with the symptoms of the menopause that manifest themselves from the outset, there is an associated disorder whose implications for their future lives are so great that it needs special consideration.

This disorder is osteoporosis which leads to a reduction in both the amount of bone tissue and the strength of it, thereby creating an abnormal susceptibility to fracture.

It is almost impossible to underestimate the potential disastrous effect that osteoporosis can have on postmenopausal women. Although in itself it is not a fatal disease it is nevertheless responsible for thousands of deaths each year as women die following fractures which resulted from bone loss.

The following statistics will give an indication of the size of the problem:

- It has been estimated that about 50 per cent of women will suffer a bone fracture resulting from osteoporosis in their lifetime, this figure including all kinds of fractures, including those of the vertebra and the wrist. More specific is the data for femoral neck fracture (that is a break in the upper part of the femur, the 'thigh bone' that links the knee joint to the pelvis) and this occurs in 12 per cent of women under the age of 85 in England and Wales, according to the *Office of Health Economics*.
- Approximately one in five of women who suffer a femoral neck fracture will die as a direct result of that injury and the associated

death rate within a year – from blood clots, pneumonia, stroke and infection – has been put as high as 50 per cent. Even for survivors, the other consequences of hip fracture can also be severe as on the average they will need to stay in hospital for about a month. Additionally, it has been estimated that only between a quarter and a half of the women who survive are likely to regain most of their mobility. This means that many will have a permanent disability which will force them to go into long-term care although previously they had been able to lead independent lives.

- While it is, of course, impossible to estimate what this means in terms of individual suffering and misery, some idea of the scope of the problem is revealed by the fact that in England and Wales there are more than 60,000 cases of hip fracture every year.
- It has been estimated that the victims of osteoporosis-linked fractures fill up to half of the orthopaedic beds in some general hospitals and that the cost of their treatment in Britain is in excess of £65 million a year.

The purpose of the above is not to frighten, but to make it abundantly clear that osteoporosis is a disorder that needs to be considered by every woman and one which she needs to take into account very seriously as she reaches her menopausal years.

THE LINK BETWEEN OSTEOPOROSIS AND THE MENOPAUSE

To clarify how the menopause can affect bone loss, it is useful first to understand how bone is made up. Bones have an outer membrane – called the *peristoneum* and made of fibrous tissue – below which lies the *compact bone*, also known as the *cortical layer*. Yet further below this is the *trabecular layer* made of so-called ‘spongy’ bone. The leg and arm bones, which are the ones most susceptible to fracture, contain but little trabecular matter except at the ends and have hollow spaces in their length which are filled with fatty marrow. In some bones, such as those in the wrist and the vertebrae, the space doesn’t contain marrow but is instead filled with trabecular bone.

Bone is made up of about one third of *collagen* (the matrix) and two thirds of minerals, the main component of which is *calcium*. It is when this calcium is lost that the bone becomes brittle and more likely to fracture under stress.

The skeleton throughout life is consistently undergoing processes of damage and repair as well as growth. These processes are controlled, among other factors, by *bone active hormones*. Oestrogen and progesterone act on the oesteoblast cells which help lay down the matrix of the bone – that is the collagen – and also affect the bone's ability to accept calcium. Broadly speaking, it can be said that oestrogen in sufficient quantities prevents the 'resorption' (that is the breakdown) of bone while progesterone helps the formation of bone.

It is hardly surprising then that when the supply of both oestrogen and progesterone declines with the menopause this in turn can profoundly affect the bones. First of all, there's a loss of efficiency in the process of bone repair, meaning that the body loses more bone than it is capable of replacing, and, secondly, ovarian failure leads to an increase in the rate of excretion of bone calcium via the urine. As collagen and mineral levels reduce, there is an accompanying reduction in bone mass – thereby making them weaker and more likely to fracture.

Summing it up, it can be safely said that postmenopausal osteoporosis is at least partly a hormone deficiency disease.

For many women, the loss of bone mass can start as early as at the age of 35 when it is comparatively slow at first. Initially, the loss is mainly of trabecular bone and this may reach a rate of three to five per cent a year by the time of the menopause and will continue at this rate for up to another ten years after which it slows down. The loss of cortical bone tends to start somewhat later, usually around the age of 45 and reaches a rate of two to three per cent a year until the mid sixties when it, too, slows down.

There are substantial individual variations in the amount of bone that is lost and while it can be difficult to predict to what extent a particular person may be affected eventually, there are certain factors which have been established as creating greater risk of osteoporosis and these include:

- *Colour of skin* – the fairer you are, the greater the likely risk.
- *Racial origin* – you're most likely to be at risk if your ancestors came from Northern Europe and less so if they were from Africa or the Mediterranean.
- *Low body mass* – the smaller you are and the less you weigh, the greater the risk, because that means you're small-boned and have less bone mass to lose in the first instance.
- *Lifestyle* – both cigarette smoking and a high alcohol intake increase risk as does a high intake of caffeine.
- *Your age at the menopause* – a premature menopause, whether resulting from natural or surgical causes, worsens the odds.

Further factors that increase risk from osteoporosis are: *Illnesses* – those who have suffered from rheumatoid arthritis, diabetes requiring insulin, thyroid problems, anorexia nervosa; *the taking of certain drugs* – steroids, thyroxine, cortico-steroids; also the long-term low intake of calcium; *other existing disease of the bones* or a family history of osteoporosis. *A sedentary lifestyle* has also been found to contribute to risk because physical activity helps build bone mass.

PREDICTING THE RISK OF BONE FRACTURE

Merely because a woman might fall into one or more of the above groups doesn't, of course, necessarily mean that she will develop osteoporosis to a severe or dangerous level. However, it does mean that her chances of this happening may be considerably higher than the average and that therefore it might be wise for her to consider making such changes to her lifestyle as she can to lower the risk.

Apart from that, it is now possible to identify those who have reduced bone density mineral content by using recently developed screening techniques, such as *quantitative computed tomography*, *dual absorptionmetry*, *single photon absorptionmetry* and – the newest of the lot – *dual X-ray energy absorptionmetry*. Such screening is, however, still very expensive and only available in a few centres and it is likely to be many years before resources will be sufficiently available to make mass population screening a possibility.

While screening is for the time being only likely to be used within the National Health Service for what have already been identified as extremely high risk cases, it is also available in certain private clinics.

HOW OSTEOPOROSIS CAN BE PREVENTED

The key to avoiding osteoporosis lies in prevention rather than cure as bone mass that has been lost cannot, broadly speaking, be replaced. So the thing to do is to avoid that loss in the first instance.

Obviously, there is nothing that a woman can do about some of the pre-disposing factors listed earlier. Others – such as lack of exercise, smoking, calcium intake – can be corrected to a point. Nevertheless, after all these things have been done, the greatest hope for avoiding osteoporosis lies in Hormone Replacement Therapy. As explained earlier, the loss of bone mass goes hand-in-hand with the reduced supply of oestrogen and progesterone during the menopause and there is now clear evidence that HRT, by replacing or supplementing hormones, can cut down the rate of loss.

HRT as a whole is covered in depth in the last two chapters of this book, but here are the key points about how it relates to osteoporosis:

- It is important that treatment should begin as soon as possible after the menopause – of course, some women will already have been receiving HRT sooner than that to relieve perimenopausal symptoms.
- Both oestrogen and progestogen have been found successfully to prevent or reduce bone loss.
- The minimum oestrogen dose that is recommended to protect the skeleton and prevent fractures is 0.625 mg of conjugated equine oestrogen or 2 mg of oestradiol. Larger doses may be indicated for some women.
- While it is generally assumed that bone loss cannot be reversed,

recent studies have suggested that an increase of two to three per cent a year in bone mass may be obtained with certain HRT combinations, these including unopposed oestrogen, and oestrogen combined with progestogen.

- The protection that HRT provides will only last as long as the treatment continues. Therefore it is generally recommended that if the prevention of bone loss is one of the major objectives of the HRT regimen it should be continued as long as possible, extending many years beyond the menopause itself if there are no contra-indications to such a long-term strategy.

CALCIUM AND NUTRITION

Although there are some differences of opinion among experts about the exact role that calcium – either as part of your normal diet or taken as a supplement – can play in preventing or reducing osteoporosis, there is agreement that you should ensure that you are at least getting the minimum requirement. And the recommended daily allowance (RDA) of calcium is:

Premenopausal women: 1000 mg
Perimenopausal women: 1200 mg
Postmenopausal women: 1400 mg

One of the reasons why the RDA increases with age is that the postmenopausal woman will absorb calcium less efficiently from the intestine.

Surveys have shown that the calcium intake of the average British woman is between 500 to 800 mg, far short of the RDAs, and this lack of calcium may be one of the reasons why osteoporosis is so prevalent. Naturally enough, one of the things that matters is your average calcium intake throughout your life and in particular during the stage when the bones were still growing. Although bringing up your calcium intake to the recommended level once the menopause has begun will be helpful, it won't be nearly as beneficial as having done so earlier.

Dietary supplements can be useful for it has been found that calcium is absorbed nearly as well in this way as it is from natural foods. There are many kinds of calcium supplements on the market and the important thing to check is how much elemental calcium each tablet actually contains. For example, a 600 mg tablet of calcium carbonate will yield 40 per cent of calcium or 240 mg; on the other hand, a 600 mg tablet of calcium lactate will only contain 13 per cent of calcium and therefore provide a mere 88 mg of it.

In order to absorb calcium properly the body also needs vitamin D and that is why some calcium supplements also include this. However, too much vitamin D can have the opposite effect in that it can increase the amount of calcium that is excreted. Generally speaking, most people, except perhaps the housebound, will get enough vitamin D from sunlight and there shouldn't be a need to supplement this.

If you feel that your diet is short on calcium and you wish to take supplements, your best bet is to talk either to your doctor or your pharmacist who will be able to advise you as to which product is most likely to serve your particular needs in a cost-effective way.

There are many foods which are rich in calcium and that, of course, is doubtlessly the best way to ensure that your supply is adequate. Here is a list of some of the best sources with the amount of calcium shown for a 100 g quantity – that being roughly equivalent to 3.5 ounces: Cheddar cheese (800 mg of calcium), semi-skimmed milk (729 mg), full-cream milk (702 mg), cheese flan (260 mg), milk chocolate (220 mg), muesli (190 mg), tinned sardines in oil (550 mg), canned pilchards (300 mg), raw broccoli (100 mg), dried figs (280 mg).

However, even if your daily intake of calcium is adequate, you can nullify this if you use too much salt which, in excess, causes an increased loss of sodium from the kidneys and this, in turn, is accompanied by an increased loss of calcium. It has been estimated that the loss rate begins to increase when the intake of salt is more than 5 g – or about a teaspoonful – a day. So there is little point in going on a calcium-rich diet or taking supplements if you don't at the same time also control your salt intake to keep it within safe limits.

The recommended daily intake is 500 mg of sodium which will be found in 1.25 g of salt. Ways of reducing your salt intake include: not adding salt to foods, avoiding convenience foods, which usually have a high salt content, avoiding baked goods made with baking powder.

While correct dieting cannot by itself guarantee that you will never suffer from osteoporosis, it can nevertheless considerably improve the odds in your favour by ensuring that your bones are as strong as they can be before the menopause starts.

8 The Menopause Doesn't Have To Be A Misery

The previous chapters have concentrated heavily on all the things that can go wrong during the menopause and the various symptoms that are linked with it. While it is true that the menopausal years can be a miserable time for many women, there is little need for it to actually be so . . . providing they seek and receive the help that is appropriate to their particular circumstances. How to avoid the menopause being a misery is what most of the remainder of this book is devoted to.

Essentially the help that is available falls into two distinct categories: those things that you can do for yourself and those where you need the help and advice of others, including doctors. We will begin by looking at the various kinds of self-help strategies that are available.

COPING WITH STRESS

Just about everyone suffers from stress at one time or another, and the menopause, particularly when it first manifests itself, is a time when stress levels are likely to be particularly high.

Stress in itself is not injurious to your health; in fact, up to a certain point it can be positively beneficial as it helps you set and attain new goals. However, if the amount of stress you're undergoing is well beyond your personal tolerance level – and these vary greatly from person to person – and this persists for some length of time, it can lead to the creation of anxiety and even depression. It follows therefore that the trick is to have just enough stress to keep you motivated, but not so much that it becomes a burden in itself.

But how much stress is enough – or, for that matter, how much is too much? There is a rather wonderful schedule called the *'Holmes-Rahe Life Stress Inventory'* which allocates a set number of points to various events as an indication of the degree of stress they cause. For example, the death of a spouse is set at 100 points while pregnancy rates a mere forty. The inventory does not list the menopause as such and the nearest thing to it is perhaps 'major personal illness or injury' which scores 53 points, somewhere between the death of a close family member (63 points) and being fired at work (50 points).

While it may be difficult to establish just how stressful the menopause actually is, there is no doubt that it does almost invariably increase the stress level for all women. The important thing to remember about stress is that it becomes harmful not just when it exceeds a certain level but when that excess is maintained over a period of time. The menopause, by definition, covers a lengthy period of time, often five years and even more, which means that the stress associated with it is always there, underlying the additional stress that may be caused by other unconnected events during that time. It is this combination of various stress factors that may push the total beyond a given person's tolerance level.

There's a three-point strategy you can follow to help reduce stress levels during the menopause:

1) You do everything you can to reduce the physical symptoms of the menopause (various ways of doing this are explained in other parts of this book).
2) During the time that the menopause is particularly stressful for you, you do your best to avoid other forms of stress. Now this may not always be possible as some stress factors are unavoidable but others may well be within your control, such as changing your job, moving house, taking on extra financial commitments.

3) Have as sensible, healthy and balanced a lifestyle as your circumstances will allow.

And, most important of all, if you think stress is getting on top of you, seek advice and help and don't just put up with more than you can reasonably cope with because you think matters will sort themselves out of their own accord.

RELAXATION TECHNIQUES

Closely allied to the subject of stress is that of relaxation because the correct use of various techniques to promote inner well-being can do wonders in coping with stress. Relaxation can also be extremely helpful in controlling and reducing the incidence of certain specific menopausal symptoms, such as palpitations, hot flushes and insomnia.

There are many different types of relaxation training and it would be beyond the scope of this book to cover them in detail. But, to get you started, here is a very simple method that can work wonders:

- Begin by lying down comfortably, either on the floor or on the bed, your head slightly supported if that feels more comfortable for you. Gradually clear your mind of any extraneous thoughts and make it as blank as possible. Then alternatively contract – that is tense – and relax various groups of muscles throughout your body. Hold each contraction for a full count of ten seconds before you consciously let go of all the tension, leaving the muscles to go completely limp. Once you've relaxed a set of muscles, leave them so and go on to the next group.
- Contract and relax the muscles in the following order: first of all, the toes, feet, calves, thighs and buttocks; then, the stomach, lower back and chest; and, finally, the shoulders, upper back, neck and face, not forgetting the forehead, nose, jaws, lips and eyes.
- When you've relaxed all your muscles, lie still for some ten minutes or so and clear your mind of all worries and problems. Feel yourself sinking down into the floor or bed as your whole body

unwinds. Some women might find that thinking about a peaceful image – such as clouds drifting across the sky or green fields – at this time will help them relax even more. Be aware of your breathing rhythm and notice how it becomes slower as you relax more deeply.

- Practise the above exercise at least once every day, more often if you have the chance, as it will probably take you a dozen or so tries before you get the hang of it and start benefiting fully.

DEALING WITH INSOMNIA

Lack of proper sleep – whether this is because it is lacking in quantity, quality, or both of these – is often one of the more debilitating symptoms of the menopause. Although the specific sleep disturbances caused by hot flushes and night sweats have been dealt with previously, here is some general advice that you might find useful in ensuring that you get a good night's sleep:

- Try to be consistent in the time you go to bed every night, thereby training your body to accept the idea of 'It's eleven o'clock, that's when I go to sleep'.
- Don't try to make up for lost sleep by staying later in bed the next morning as this will probably only make it more difficult for you to get off to sleep the following night.
- It's generally recommended that you shouldn't eat just before going to bed. However, some people do find that a light late night snack helps.
- Drinking alcohol shortly before going to bed interferes with the sleep pattern of most people. You might be the exception and you could experiment with a small nightcap and see if that helps.
- Daytime naps are the enemy of a good night's sleep. No matter how tired you might feel during the day, resist the urge to have a nap.
- If you can, stop smoking. If that's beyond you, try at least not to smoke during the last few hours before bedtime.
- A short walk in the evening might help by making you feel

physically tired and so assist in a good night's sleep.
- Avoid drinking tea or coffee late in the evening.
- Plan to have a period of quiet relaxation before going to bed.

PHYSICAL EXERCISE

Most of us are well aware that physical exercise is vital throughout life to maintain the efficiency of the heart and the cardiovascular system. What is less well known, however, is the role that the right kind of exercise can play in the maintenance of your bone mass which, of course, comes under attack from osteoporosis during the menopause. There is nevertheless a curious kind of Catch-22 situation here in that, strangely enough, being overweight can in itself provide a certain amount of protection against osteoporosis because the extra fat cells will produce additional oestrone – a weak kind of oestrogen – and this will help supplement the reduced supply of hormones from the ovaries. Despite that, the overall recommendation remains that menopausal women should strive not to be overweight because of other health considerations. There are only two ways that weight can be lost: either by taking in fewer calories or by burning off more of them.

While just about all kinds of exercise can be helpful, there are some that are best avoided during and after the menopause because the spine may have been affected by osteoporosis in its early stage. Therefore it is recommended that exercises involving great extension or flexion of the back should not be attempted because of the risk of injury to a weakened spine. Should osteoporosis have been detected as being actually present, then exercise is probably best limited to reasonably brisk walking or swimming.

On the other hand, before the menopause has begun, exercises involving the large muscle groups – that's the abdominal muscles, the back muscles, and hamstrings – are considered particularly beneficial.

Swimming, of course, is one of the best overall forms of exercise, as it provides muscle toning without undue stretching. The next best thing for most people is likely to be what is called 'structured walking', which involves dividing the time allowed for the walk, say 45 minutes, into three separate sections, each with its own specific part to play in the overall programme. What you do during the first 15 minutes or so is to warm up gradually, beginning by walking steadily but not fast and accelerating the pace until you're walking briskly. The second 15-minute segment is devoted to walking at a pace fast enough to provide aerobic and cardiovascular benefit. This is generally defined as a walk brisk enough to produce a heart rate of 200 less your age (for example, if you're 45, keep the heart rate down to 155; if you're 30, let it go up to 170, but no more). The final 15 minutes are used as a cool-down period during which you gradually reduce your pace to return to normal.

SENSIBLE DIETING

Strangely enough, there has been virtually no research into diet and the menopause except for investigations into the role of calcium in relation to osteoporosis. Yet, although the menopause hasn't been specifically identified as a cause of possible nutritional stress, this is obviously a time when it is particularly sensible to eat a well-balanced diet. That, however, leaves the question as to what exactly does a well-balanced diet consist of, a question that is likely to have many different answers depending upon who you choose to ask.

However, despite all the faddish nutritional advice which abounds wherever you look, there are certain main points upon which most authorities are in agreement. And these key facts are:

- Less than 35 per cent of your food intake energy should be supplied by dietary fat.
- Less than 10 per cent of your food intake energy should come from saturated fats.
- Broadly speaking, most people would benefit from increasing their intake of cereals and starches.
- The intake of sugar, except from milk sources, should be reduced.

- Salt consumption should be reduced.

Nutritionists are also mainly in agreement that a well-balanced diet should consist of approximately 56 per cent of carbohydrates, 14 per cent of protein, and that the total fat content – that is all forms of dietary fat, including saturated, polyunsaturated and mono-unsaturated fats – should be no more than 30 per cent. A further recommendation is that you should eat a wide variety of foods that are rich in fibre to ensure that your daily intake includes at least 25 grams of soluble and insoluble fibre for their effect in aiding digestion.

ALCOHOL INTAKE

Closely linked to nutrition is the question of alcohol intake, especially as this can also have a very specific effect on the development of osteoporosis.

First of all, it's important to be aware that alcohol is broken down in the body in a different way by women and that this means that the alcohol level to body weight ratio is higher for them than it is for men. Among other things, this means that women as a group are therefore more susceptible to alcoholism and that they should perhaps monitor their alcohol intake more carefully.

Current official advice is that women should not drink more than 14 units of alcohol in any given week and that not more than two units should be taken in a given day. To put this in perspective, all of the following represent one unit of alcohol: one glass of wine; one measure of sherry, spirits or liqueur; half a pint of beer, lager or cider; a quarter pint of strong ale or strong lager.

As far as osteoporosis is concerned, alcohol can reduce bone-forming activity – thereby reducing bone mass – by preventing calcium absorption from the bowel. So, from that point of view, an even lower intake than the limits suggested above might be wise.

LOOKING GOOD

Apart from wanting to feel physically well, women naturally also want to look their best. Unfortunately, some of the side-effects of the menopause can create very specific problems in this area. Although it is not the function of this book to provide beauty hints (there are many other books on that subject), you might find the following information useful:

SKIN CARE. There is a certain amount of disagreement about the extent to which the menopause actually affects the condition of the skin. Some authorities maintain that the reduced oestrogen creates a marked decrease in the amount of collagen in the skin, thereby reducing its elasticity, and also that the skin becomes thinner. While there is a lot of evidence to back this up and there is no doubt that this happens to a point, others say that the effect is minimal and that what really occurs is that the menopause happens to coincide with a time when the skin starts to show the results of how you've treated it throughout your life.

Skin – and facial skin in particular – is gradually weathered over the years by wind, sun and pollution, and quite naturally as a woman gets older the cumulative effects of this start to show mainly in the form of dry skin. While cosmetic preparations – despite their claims to the contrary – cannot prevent the aging of skin, the dryness of it can be alleviated to a great extent by the use of simple skin moisturisers. What the moisturiser actually does is to provide a thin waterproof layer over the skin and thereby reduces the loss of water from the skin itself. Very little – if any – of the moisturiser is actually absorbed by the skin as the very purpose of the skin is to prevent that happening. Nevertheless, moisturisers do work and can reduce or prevent drying.

HAIR CARE. Once again, the professionals are divided on the question of the extent to which the menopause affects hair condition. One authority states categorically "hair roots are affected by lack of oestrogen . . . and thicker, healthier hair is another benefit to be gained from oestrogen", while another says "hair does not change significantly after the menopause, although it may become thinner with age".

So the question remains: is the thinning of hair that is noted by many women in their fifties just part of the normal aging process or is it mainly due to reduced oestrogen levels caused by the menopause? Part of the answer to this might lie in the experiences of women who have had Hormone Replacement Therapy and who in many instances have reported that thickening of previously thinning hair was one of the side-benefits of treatment.

Perhaps for most women the question of why the hair thins around the time of the menopause is of academic interest only and their prime concern is what can be done to minimise the effect that the thinning has on their appearance. Apart from considering HRT (and the decision to take this treatment is naturally based on more fundamental health issues), the best general advice is to put the matter in the hands of the most knowledgeable hairdresser you can find who will be able to advise you as to what hairstyles, tints and colourings will be most effective for you. Should you have specific problems, it may be advisable to consult a qualified trichologist.

9 How Others Can Help You

The previous chapter has been primarily concerned with the various things you can do yourself to make your transition through the menopause easier. We will now look at the various kinds of help that are available from outside sources, whether this be in the form of medical advice or treatment, drugs and other preparations, or alternative therapies.

YOUR FAMILY DOCTOR

The views and opinions held by your doctor about the menopause can have a profound effect upon how easily you will be able to cope with its various effects. Unfortunately it must be said that many doctors – and that also includes a goodly number of those who are women themselves – are still inclined to be somewhat dismissive when confronted with a patient whose symptoms are all clearly of a menopausal nature.

This lack of proper counselling was highlighted by a recent postal survey conducted by the *Amarant Trust* among more than 3,000 women which found that overall 44.5 per cent of women were dissatisfied with the duration of their initial consultation, this figure referring to consultations with either general practitioners or specialist consultants. Of those seen only by GPs, the percentage of dissatisfied patients rose to nearly 80 per cent.

Another set of statistics from the same survey also showed that family doctors ranked a poor second (at just under 20 per cent) as the most commonly used source of information about Hormone Replacement Therapy, with written material in the form of newspapers or magazines coming out at the top with a score of 50 per cent.

These figures clearly underline that there is still a vast gulf to be bridged between patients and their family doctors. Having said that, there is also little doubt that the situation is improving and that more and more family doctors are taking a greater interest in the menopause and that there is also a great deal more information about it appearing in medical journals.

In the meantime, however, it is only all too possible that a patient seeking advice from her doctor may not get all that much help as some are obviously either unwilling or unable to devote time to counselling or providing information about the menopause. This is what some women had to say about what happened when they first saw their doctor about menopausal problems:

"I told him how the frequency of my hot flushes was making it very difficult for me at work. He just looked at me and said, 'Well, that's just one of those things you have to put up with as you get older'."

"When I asked my doctor whether HRT might be a good idea for me as my mother and aunt had both had hip fractures in their sixties, he said that there was still a lot of doubt about how much good hormone replacement really did."

"After I had outlined all my symptoms – all the classical menopausal ones like hot flushes, night sweats, unpredictable periods – he prescribed a mild tranquilliser, saying, 'That will stop you worrying too much about things'."

"My doctor is a very good one, but I swear that he actually became embarrassed when I began to talk about the menopause."

So what are your options if your doctor is somewhat like the ones mentioned above? You have four possible choices:

1) You can change doctors altogether, but that is a fairly complicated procedure at the best of times and you also have to be sure that you're not jumping from the frying pan into the fire by trying to find out in advance what

your new doctor's views are on the menopause.

2) If your doctor is part of a large practice with several partners, you may be able to find out from the receptionist which of the other partners may be more sympathetic. By the way, don't assume that a woman doctor will necessarily serve you better as other people's experiences have shown this to be by no means always the case.
3) You can ask your doctor to refer you to a gynaecologist which he will almost be duty bound to do.
4) You can ask to be referred to a special menopause clinic. Unfortunately such clinics, which are usually attached to the larger teaching hospitals, are still comparatively few in number. (You will find a list of the main ones in Appendix A at the back of this book.)

The above, of course, refers to your options within the National Health Service. If you're willing – and able – to pay for treatment there are other possibilities, such as seeing a gynaecologist privately (a referral letter from your doctor may still be needed by some of these and this will definitely be necessary if you intend to reclaim your costs from a private medical insurance scheme such as BUPA or Private Patients Plan).

While the above may have given the impression that some doctors fall short of what is required of them by menopausal women, it must also be pointed out that there are many family doctors who do provide an excellent service. A relatively new innovation is the provision of a menopause clinic within the 'Well Woman Clinics' operated by some of the larger practices with one or more partners specialising in that area of medicine.

Finally, a word of advice. If, for good reason, you're not happy with what your doctor is doing – or perhaps not doing – to help you with your menopausal problems, don't just accept this and keep putting up with the symptoms. In the first instance, attempt to convince your own doctor that your situation deserves attention; if that doesn't work, do seek advice elsewhere.

As to what your doctor can do to help, that will vary considerably according to the severity and scope of the symptoms. Hormone Replacement Therapy – which is covered in detail in the next chapter – is but one of the possibilities and not always the one of choice. Other treatments which may prove helpful include:

ANTIDEPRESSANTS AND TRANQUILLISERS. Although these will not deal with the root-cause of certain menopausal problems, they can be helpful in the short-term to alleviate some symptoms. However, both of these require constant supervision as the risk of dependency and/or abuse is only too real.

CLONIDINE HYDROCHLORIDE. This is a drug that is also used to prevent recurrent migraine and vascular headaches and it has been found helpful in preventing or reducing menopausal hot flushes. But Clonidine Hydrochloride will not relieve any of the other menopausal symptoms resulting from reduced hormone levels. The usual dosage is 50 micrograms taken twice a day. There are some contra-indications to this treatment as it can aggravate depression or produce insomnia, both of which, of course, are also often part of the menopausal syndrome.

VITAMIN B6 (PYRIDOXINE). Although you can buy this for yourself across the counter in pharmacies or health food shops, you'd be wise to consult your doctor before doing so. Vitamin B6 is most likely to be helpful in combating those menopausal symptoms which closely resemble those of Premenstrual Syndrome and, in fact, the *British National Formulary* suggests that a daily dose of 50 to 100 mg may be prescribed for this purpose. However, various side-effects – including skin rashes, undue sensitivity of the skin, and weakness of muscles – have been reported when B6 has been taken in high dosages over a lengthy period of time.

VITAMIN E. This vitamin has been credited by many women with helping to relieve hot flushes and night sweats although there is no medical evidence to substantiate that claim and the *Committee on Safety of Medicines* states 'Vitamin E has been tried for various conditions, but there is no scientific evidence of its value'. This vitamin should not be taken without first consulting your doctor if you have heart problems, diabetes or high blood pressure. Additionally, you must bear in mind that Vitamin E also contains a small amount of oestrogens which means that if oestrogens are contra-indicated in your case so will be the vitamin. If you do decide to try it, begin with a very small dose at first, such as 100 international units every day for a month or so and see if it brings you any benefit.

OIL OF EVENING PRIMROSE. This is now a very popular remedy for PMS symptoms and is also taken by many women to reduce menopausal side-effects. The seed oil of the evening primrose plant (Oenothera biennis) is a rich source of *Gamma Linolenic Acid (GLA)* which is converted in the body to *prostaglandins* which influence hormone relationships and therefore it is possible that the GLA may help correct hormone imbalance. Dosage is variable, but one 500 mg capsule taken once or twice a day might be a good way to start, increasing this if need be after a month or so. Although there are no specific contra-indications for this preparation, it is best taken with food as it has been known otherwise to create nausea. Other rich sources of GLA are sunflower, safflower and corn oils.

GINSENG. Ginseng can contain small amounts of oestrogen, so don't take this if oestrogen is contra-indicated for you. Asthmatics should also be careful of taking ginseng because of its histamine properties, and if you have any doubts, check first with your doctor. Once again, this is one of those popular remedies for menopausal problems – used, in particular, for the relief of hot flushes, headaches and palpitations – which although credited with great potency by many women still lacks a formal scientific endorsement. Having said that, it might be worth a try as so many claim that it has done wonders for them. You can get ginseng – apparently the Siberian variety is better for menopausal problems than the Korean one – from health food shops and the recommended daily dosage is around 500 mg of the dried root. It is also available in capsule form.

OTHER HERBAL PREPARATIONS. Although once again not endorsed by scientific evidence, there are several other natural remedies that many women have found to help relieve menopausal symptoms. Included among these are *liquorice root*, *female ginseng* (also known as *tan kwai*), *sarsaparilla*, *gotu kola*, *fenugreek*, as well as *camomile and other herbal teas*. While these are freely available from many chemists as well as health food shops, it must be kept in mind that they can nevertheless cause side-effects and you'd always be wise to try them out in small amounts in the first instance.

ALTERNATIVE THERAPIES

There is a vast range of alternative therapies which can offer help with certain menopausal symptoms. Which of these to try is a matter of individual choice, but all the ones listed below have their ardent supporters. One note of caution, however: while alternative therapies may be suitable for the relief and treatment of certain recurrent symptoms – such as headaches, feelings of anxiety, hot flushes and night sweats – you should always consult your doctor beforehand to ensure that a proper medical diagnosis is made first. You should also seek medical advice immediately if you develop any serious symptoms, such as vaginal bleeding after intercourse, or find any breast irregularities.

ACUPUNCTURE. This is one part of the ancient Oriental medical system developed in China. The therapy works by using needles – or other objects – to stimulate specific points on the body to create changes in other parts of the body. One of the aims of this system is to rebalance forces and thereby improve health.

Acupuncturists believe in the Chinese philosophy that states there is a life force – called chi – which is composed of negative and positive flows of energy, respectively known as yin and yang, which course throughout the body along channels which are known as meridians. Diseases and pain are seen as the results of an interruption or an imbalance in these energy flows.

Acupuncture is perhaps one of the best-known forms of alternative medicine in the West and it has a long record of being particularly effective in the relief of pain. It is also frequently used by doctors. As with so many other forms of alternative medicine, it is best to consult a qualified practitioner and a list of registered acupuncturists can be obtained from: *The British Medical Acupuncture Society, Newton House, Newton Lane, Lower Whitley, Warrington, Cheshire WA4 4JA, 092-573 727.*

ACUPRESSURE. The principle underlying this therapy is essentially the same as that for acupuncture except that the points in the body are massaged with the finger or the thumb instead of using needles. One of the advantages of this is that a patient may well be able to perform this massage herself. Most acupuncture practitioners also offer acupressure treatment.

HOMOEOPATHY. This is a system of medicine developed by Samuel Hahnemann in the late 1700s and is based on the twin principles that *'like cures like'* and *'less is more'*. This is reflected in the homoeopathic belief that symptoms are signs produced by the body's effort to resist or throw off disease.

Homoeopaths claim that the body can cope with most illnesses and that it is the doctor's job to help strengthen the body's innate ability to heal itself. Treatment usually consists of extremely small doses of preparations, either as tablets or as liquids, made from natural substances and originating from herbal, animal, mineral and metallic sources. One of the guiding principles of homoeopathy is 'Minimal Dose' and in practice this means that the remedies are prescribed in a form that is so diluted that none of the original substance can still be detected in the final mixture. This, of course, raises the question of how can a remedy possibly work if there is nothing – or very little – left of the original substance? Most practitioners admit that they don't actually know. Despite this, homoeopathy has been proven time and time again to provide results under the most stringent test conditions. Many medically-qualified doctors also practice homoeopathy.

You can get more information about homoeopathy from: *The British Homoeopathic Association, 27a Devonshire Street, London W1N 1RJ, 071-935 2163; or the Hahnemann Society, Hahnemann*

House, 2 Powis Place, Great Ormond Street, London WC1N 3HT, 071-837 3297.

AROMATHERAPY. The basic principle of this therapy is the use of *essential oils* – derived from wild or cultivated plants, trees, herbs and fruit – to restore the body's natural functions and rhythms. These essences can be used in several different ways: as compresses, in baths, as inhalants, and for massages. One of the oils used is that of sage which contains an oestrogen and native American women have traditionally used this herb to help control menstruation.

A word of caution: some of the oils can be poisonous except in the very smallest amounts, so it is essential that aromatherapy is supervised by a qualified person. You can get a list of registered aromatherapists by sending an SAE to: *International Federation of Aromatherapists, 4 Eastmearn Road, West Dulwich, London SE21 8HA.* Note, however, that this is a representative, not licensing, organisation.

REFLEXOLOGY. This is a technique that works by stroking or applying pressure to one part of the body, usually the feet or hands, to create changes elsewhere and, in particular, to stimulate the body's own ability to heal itself. Results vary greatly, but treatment is unlikely to be harmful and has been found effective by many. You can get more information from: *The British School of Reflexology, 92 Sheering Road, Old Harlow, Essex CM17 0JW, 0279-429 060.*

NATUROPATHY, also known as **NATUROPATHIC MEDICINE.** This combines a wide variety of natural therapeutic and healing techniques and can perhaps best be described as a mixture of traditional folk wisdom and modern medicine. One of the underlying principles of this therapy is that the root of all disease is the accumulation of waste products and toxins within the body, this usually resulting from a deficient lifestyle. Naturopaths also believe that the human body has the wisdom and the power to heal itself, providing that we enhance rather than interfere with this power. In actual treatment, naturopathy relies heavily on diet management techniques and herbal preparations. You can get more information from: *The British Naturopathic and*

Osteopathic Association, Frazer House, 6 Netherhall Gardens, London NW3 5RR, 071-435 8728.

BACH FLOWER REMEDIES. Dr Edward Bach was a homoeopathic physician and bacteriologist who created Flower Remedies in the 1930s to treat emotional imbalances. You can get more information from: *The Edward Bach Centre, Mount Vernon, Sotwell, Wallingford, Oxon OX10 0PZ.*

HYPNOSIS AND HYPNOTHERAPY. The effects of hypnosis are well documented and its use is nowadays quite common by the medical profession for all sorts of purposes, including inducing anaesthesia. In recent years, it has also been used by an increasing number of psychotherapists to allay fears, reduce anxiety and treat depressive states.

Hypnosis is essentially the use of the power of suggestion; whether that suggestion comes from the hypnotist or from the patient herself. It has proven itself particularly effective in treating psychosomatic conditions, such as skin disorders, certain types of asthma, migraine and so on, but has also proven itself in reducing the effect of vasomotor symptoms common during the menopause. Sources of information include: *The British Society of Hypnotherapists, 37 Orbain Road, Fulham, London SW6 7JZ*; *The International Association of Hypnotherapists, 1 Lowther Gardens, Bournemouth, Dorset BH8 8NH*; and *The World Federation of Hypnotherapists, Belmont Centre, 46 Belmont Road, Ramsgate, Kent CT11 7QG.*

YOGA. This well-known discipline consists of two separate yet inter-linked components: firstly, there's a series of static or stretching exercises and breathing practices; secondly, there is a meditation discipline which aims to reach a state of peace and harmony in the inner self.

At the physical level, yoga can be extremely effective as a way of relieving stress levels and as such may help with psychological problems associated with the menopause. The meditation techniques may also be found beneficial for those suffering from stress.

While nearly all yoga exercises are safe for a moderately fit person, there are some that produce too much strain on the bones for women who suffer from osteoporosis. All but the simplest exercises should therefore only be undertaken under the supervision of a qualified teacher. And, if you have osteoporosis, do tell the teacher so beforehand.

For more information contact: *The British Wheel of Yoga, 1 Hamilton Place, Boston Road, Sleaford, Lincolnshire NG34 7ES, 0529-306851.*

SELF-HELP GROUPS

In recent years, many 'self-help' groups have been set up in various parts of the country by women getting together to exchange views about the menopause. It is in the nature of such grass-roots groups that they may come and go in a given locality and as such there is no national organisation nor central register for them. Although difficult to locate, these menopause groups can nevertheless be extremely useful for the mutual support and exchange of information they can offer.

If you want to find out whether there is a group of that kind in your area, the first place to ask is at your doctor's surgery. If that doesn't yield results, ask at your local hospital's gynaecology department, your local Well Woman Clinic or Family Planning Centre. Alternatively, your local library may have details in their files on local organisations.

If you're unable to locate a group, you just might consider the possibility of setting one up yourself. You could do this by placing a small ad in your local paper – or writing a letter to its editor – to locate other women who might be interested.

10 How Hormone Replacement Therapy Works

Although there have been numerous brief references to Hormone Replacement Therapy – also known as 'HRT' – in previous chapters of this book, a full explanation of it has been reserved until now so that all the salient facts about it can be easily found in one place.

As its name implies, the purpose of HRT is to replace the hormones whose natural level of production drops and eventually disappears when a woman becomes perimenopausal. The word 'replace' is very important in this context because in that respect HRT is very different from the contraceptive pill which provides additional hormones instead of artificially continuing a supply.

This distinction between 'adding' or 'replacing' hormones becomes very relevant when considering whether HRT is a 'natural' thing to do, a subject upon which many women hold widely opposing views. While that argument is not likely to be settled in the near future, it is clear however that continuing – albeit artificially – the supply of a hormone that the body had previously manufactured for itself, is more natural than to increase substantially an already adequate supply.

The purpose of HRT is essentially two-fold:

1) Reducing the incidence and severity of the various symptoms, linked to the falling hormone levels, which are part of the menopause by providing replacement hormones.
2) Helping to prevent certain of the problems – such as osteoporosis – which are often part of the postmenopausal pattern.

The idea of HRT is hardly new and in one form or another has been with us for about 40 years, with some of the forerunners of the current therapy being known as ORT or ERT, this standing for 'oestrogen replacement therapy', with how you chose to spell oestrogen determining the initials. Even well before that there were various experiments and as early as 1908, one researcher claimed that using extracts from various glands – thyroid, ovarian and parotid – had given promising results in reducing menopausal symptoms.

Although HRT has nowadays gained acceptance from the medical community, it was not always so and in its initial days there was strong resistance to it from many doctors. Part of this may have stemmed from innate conservatism, but some of this resistance may also have been the result of the manner in which HRT was originally promoted in the United States, where it was hailed as a panacea that would ensure eternal youth, vigour and beauty for all women who took it.

The cause of HRT was also set back in 1975 when there was a scare that claimed that it could cause cancer. This was at a time when oestrogen was used alone without the addition of progesterone and that single hormone replacement therapy did indeed at times create a condition known as *hyperplasia*, a build-up of the lining of the womb. Although hyperplasia was not cancerous, it could – if neglected – create conditions that could lead to uterine cancer. Although remote, there was indeed a link between ORT and cancer and, not surprisingly, confidence in the new treatment suffered a setback.

Since those early days, the newer and more effective forms of HRT have become firmly established as a treatment that offers a multitude of benefits with a minimum of risk for most patients. Despite that there are startling differences in the extent to which it is used by women in different countries: in America and Canada, where the medical profession heartily endorses it and even could be said to be promoting it, something like 80 per cent of women presenting menopausal symptoms will receive HRT. In the United Kingdom, however, only about ten per cent of those likely to benefit from it are currently receiving HRT.

Why is there such a difference? No one knows for sure, but one factor that is obviously at work here is that British doctors are traditionally more conservative in prescribing 'new' treatments than their North American counterparts. Doubtlessly the other factor is that British women themselves are generally not as aware of what HRT is and what it can do for them and therefore don't ask their doctors for it. There is evidence, however, to show that things are changing rapidly in this country and the number of women taking HRT is increasing all the time.

Although HRT is unquestionably of great benefit to most women – one book described it as 'the greatest treasure of a middle-aged woman's life, I've reached fifty but feel twenty . . .' – it is not suitable for all women. Essentially there are two main reasons why HRT may not be indicated:

1) Something like 15 per cent of women find that they either have or develop an intolerance to HRT and as a result experience symptoms like fluid retention, headaches, weight gain, as well as symptoms similar to those of premenstrual tension.
2) HRT can create additional risks if certain other conditions exist. The following are judged to be absolute contra-indications for HRT: endometrial or breast cancer, pregnancy, undiagnosed vaginal bleeding, certain types of lumps in the breast, severe thromboembolism. There are other conditions which are seen as relative contra-indications – which means that HRT might be prescribed, but only after very careful consideration of all the factors involved – and these include varicose veins, diabetes, liver or gall-bladder disease, fibroids, a history of endometrial hyperplasia, benign breast disease, certain types of thrombosis, and otosclerosis (which is a deterioration of the inner part of the ear, usually associated with advancing years).

Incidentally, you may have been told that you should not have HRT if you're a smoker. That, strictly speaking, isn't so because smoking, although increasing your risks of heart and circulatory diseases as well as those of throat and lung cancer, does not increase any of the risks of HRT itself. What smoking does do is to increase the rate of destruction of oestrogen and thereby make HRT less effective. There is, however, another very good reason why smokers should be encouraged to stop in their middle years which has nothing to do with HRT as such and is simply that there are many diseases whose risk factor increases around the time of the menopause, whether or not you're having HRT.

So, although there are good reasons why some women shouldn't have HRT, what then are the benefits that it can produce for the rest?

There's no short answer to that question because although the medical literature abounds with the results of various surveys there is quite often a lack of consistency in the findings as to the extent that various menopausal symptoms responded to HRT. There is, however, a much broader agreement concerning the main symptoms that were likely to respond well to HRT and these included: hot flushes, night sweats, insomnia, headaches, panic attacks, palpitations, mood changes, anxiety and irritability as well as certain types of depression, poor memory or concentration, loss of confidence, painful intercourse, loss of interest in sex, increased urinary frequency or urgency, thinning of the skin and hair, and painful joints.

It's a lengthy list indeed as it includes just about every unpleasant menopausal symptom and you could be forgiven for thinking that HRT is indeed a wonder treatment. However, you should bear in mind that while HRT, for example, has proved beneficial in treating depression, that doesn't mean that it has cleared up all instances of depression. The same thing goes for the other symptoms on the list – in most instances HRT will help, but it certainly will not always help all patients with all symptoms.

As a generality, as specific results can vary tremendously from patient to patient, HRT will do particularly well in relieving the vasomotor symptoms of the menopause, that is hot flushes, night sweats and so on. It will also be quite effective in dealing with the milder forms of psychological problems providing that these stem originally from hormonal imbalance. Genito-urinary symptoms can also be expected to respond favourably, but the individual variations may be greater as is the case for other, less clearly defined, problems such as thin hair and skin, aches and pains in joints and so on.

Apart from its effects on the symptoms listed above, there are also two other excellent reasons why HRT, if suitable, is to be recommended:

1) It has been shown to reduce the rate of bone loss (osteoporosis) which otherwise would result from the lowered levels of both oestrogen and progesterone during the perimenopausal and postmenopausal years.
2) It reduces the risk of cardiovascular disease – 'cardioprotective' is the medical term for this action – by, so it is believed, promoting beneficial changes in cholesterol levels.

Although the potential benefits of HRT are numerous, there are however some drawbacks. For many women the chief one of these is that the kind of HRT mainly prescribed nowadays, combining oestrogen with progestogen, will produce 'monthly bleeds', these being rather like menstrual periods although these themselves might have stopped some time before.

The reason for adding the progestogen – which is responsible for producing the monthly bleeds – is to 'oppose' the effect of the oestrogen which – when left unopposed – can lead to excessive endometrial thickening with its attendant additional risk of eventual cancer. Of course, the addition of the progestogen is only needed by women who still have an intact uterus – should they have had a hysterectomy previously there is no need for the progestogen as there naturally is no uterine lining to be concerned about.

While most women are prepared to tolerate the unwanted side-effect of monthly bleeds – considering this a comparatively small price to pay to gain relief from menopausal symptoms – there are some who feel otherwise and may choose not to have HRT. Broadly speaking, those who find that the disadvantage of monthly bleeds outweighs the benefits of HRT tend to fall into one of two groups:

1) Women whose menopausal problems have caused them but little concern and therefore will quite reasonably conclude that the re-establishment of monthly bleeds is more trouble than the relatively minor benefits they may derive from HRT treatment. It must, however, be pointed out that this assessment generally doesn't fully take into account the potential long-term benefits of HRT, including its effect in reducing the risk of osteoporosis.
2) Older women – who often will have asked for long-term HRT in the first instance mainly to guard against osteoporosis – can find the recurrence of monthly bleeds, especially if they had been free of these for many years, unacceptable and they may stop HRT.

Although the nuisance of monthly bleeds remains part and parcel of HRT for most women currently, there is every likelihood that in the relatively near future it may be possible to eliminate these with new combinations of oestrogens and progestogens. These treatments – known as *'continuous combined' regimens* – consist of taking both oestrogen and progestogen daily. Early reports of these new preparations have been encouraging although some 10 per cent of the patients still reported bleeding during the fourth month of starting them. Additionally, there is still a question mark about the long-term safety of this approach and, for the time being, it is recommended that women on such a regimen should have regular sampling of the endometrium by biopsy.

While further data is awaited on the 'continuous combined' treatment outlined above, the main form of HRT being prescribed currently is what is called *'cyclic opposed'*. In that phrase, 'cyclic' means that the treatment is taken over successive cycles of 28 days and 'opposed' denotes that the oestrogen is 'opposed' by the addition of progestogen for some of the time. This kind of regimen closely imitates the natural rise and fall of hormonal levels in non-menopausal women and has been shown to reduce the risk of endometrial cancer to a lower level than that of the untreated population.

Apart from the different types of regimens, there are also several kinds of HRT and methods of administration. The oestrogens may be either synthetic or natural, the latter being of animal origin with pregnant mares providing the most common source. While the natural oestrogens are not as potent as the artificial alternatives, synthetic oestrogens are chemically quite different and usually have additional effects on liver proteins, such as creating changes in blood clotting and blood lipid levels.

Which particular form of HRT may be prescribed is likely to depend greatly upon which preparation a doctor may have found most effective for his patients in the past. This is because there is little comparative data available to date to show that one form of natural oestrogen is particularly better than another, whether the comparison is made on the basis of greater relief of symptoms, incidence of side-effects or the possibility of adverse long-term consequences.

Here is a list of some of the main HRT preparations currently available in Britain.

OPPOSED OESTROGEN TAKEN ORALLY

Oestradiol, oestriol and norethisterone acetate – consisting of human oestrogens with norethisteron acetate for 10 days. One tablet daily from a 28-day calendar dial pack.

Conjugated equine oestrogens and norgestrel – consisting of horse-derived oestrogen with norgestrel for 12 days. Presented as a blister pack requiring the taking of one tablet daily for 16 days followed by two tablets daily during the added progestogen phase.

Oestradiol valerate and dl-norgestrel – consisting of ester of human oestrogen with 10 days of dl-norgestrel. One tablet daily from a 21-day blister pack.

Metranol and norethisterone – consisting of synthetic oestrogen with 13 days of norethisterone. One tablet daily from a 28-day blister pack.

OESTROGEN ALONE TAKEN ORALLY

Conjugated equine oestrogen – consisting of a combination of oestrone, equilin, equilenin and sulphates, and oestradiol. Dose: 0.625 to 1.25 mg.

Oestrone piperazine sulphate – consisting of ester of oestrone. Dose: 1.5 mg.

Oestradiol valerate – consisting of ester of oestradiol. Dose: 1 to 2 mg.

Administration of HRT by tablets is currently the method most commonly used in Britain as well as in the United States. It has the advantage for the patient that it is convenient and the calendar type blister packs clearly show when a tablet has been taken, thereby lessening the chances of making a mistake.

A newer way of administering HRT for women where there is no need to oppose it with progestogen is by using a dermal patch which allows the absorption of oestrogen through the skin. One advantage of this method is that the hormone replacement goes directly into the circulation thereby avoiding having to go first through the liver as oral preparations do. Additionally, the skin patch method has also been found less likely to produce nausea which has been associated with oral administration. On the other hand, not all women who tried the patch considered it satisfactory with one survey finding that one in twenty users had reported skin irritation and itching caused by the adhesive on the patch, while an equal number found that the patch had loosened well before it was time to change it.

For the time being, the skin patch is only used to provide a continuous controlled supply of oestradiol and it is therefore an unopposcd regimen. In some instances, however, when the patch for one reason or another is the route of choice it may be used in conjunction with progestogen taken orally.

Another method of administering HRT is via a subcutaneous implant of oestradiol. This, too, has the advantage of by-passing the liver, but there have been problems with swings in the blood oestradiol levels so that frequent monitoring is also recommended. As this monitoring requires the patients to attend clinics for blood tests it is not surprising that implants so far have not proven as popular as other methods.

Once again, the implants – which are about the size of a small pea and are usually inserted in the fatty tissue of the abdomen or thigh under local anaesthetic – only provide oestradiol and if the uterus is present progestogens should be taken for 12 days of the month. A further possible problem with implants is that there is little that can be done, apart from giving symptomatic relief where possible, if unpleasant side-effects materialise during the useful life of the implant which is usually four to six months.

The methods above are all concerned with administering HRT in a systemic – that is generalised – way. However, hormone replacement may also be prescribed in a topical – that is local – form so that its effects will be primarily directed at a specific target area. Topical preparations are supplied as either vaginal creams or pessaries and are therefore rapidly absorbed by the surrounding tissues. The whole point of these is, of course, that they are extremely useful when atrophic vaginitis is present and requires treatment, but that other menopausal symptoms aren't presented strongly enough to warrant attention.

Although the creams and pessaries act locally, they do have an uncontrolled absorption rate which can mean that there still is a possibility of systemic side-effects. For that reason, the same contra-indications which would apply if the HRT were taken orally must still be considered.

It's clear from the above that the best method of administration in a given case is not always obvious, with the various pros and cons having to be carefully weighed up. Women will have their individual preferences as will their doctors, but there is one more factor that may influence the final decision and that is the one of likely 'compliance', this being the term used to describe the likelihood that a patient will actually take the prescription, or 'comply' with it.

Obviously, there is no chance of lack of compliance with implants.

Skin patches, on the other hand, have a somewhat mixed record as they can become detached or patients have been known to remove them if the skin became too irritated. Tablets – provided as they are in almost fool-proof packaging – usually score well in the compliance stakes, but nevertheless full compliance is by no means guaranteed. Naturally enough, the best guarantee of compliance is a well-motivated patient who fully understands that the treatment should be followed exactly as prescribed if the desired results are to be achieved.

In most cases, doctors will choose to prescribe HRT at the lowest possible dosage initially, only increasing this if the symptoms persist. Generally, this will mean that the treatment offered in the first instance will be a cyclical preparation with progestogen added for part of the cycle. Normally, the situation will be reviewed periodically when either the dosage may be changed or an alternative method considered if the original treatment is either not dealing effectively with the menopausal symptoms or if there are side-effects.

Women also naturally want to know when they should start taking HRT for the first time. Posing that question is a little bit like putting the horse before the cart as HRT will only be prescribed after they have seen their doctor – and they're not likely to have done that until they have experienced menopausal symptoms of some severity. Even then, some doctors may prefer to delay HRT for some time to find out whether the symptoms decrease or even disappear of their own accord, so it may be some time before treatment actually starts.

Incidentally, there are two types of patients for whom HRT is usually prescribed at the onset: women who have had their ovaries surgically removed for non-malignant causes (such as cysts) or who are having a premature menopause, unless, of course, there are severe contra-indications in the form of other health factors.

For most women, however, HRT will start once their menopausal symptoms have reached the stage where they have sought help for them. That is likely to be somewhere between four and two years before menstruation stops completely as this is the time span where the hormone supply from the ovaries begins to drop off considerably and create the symptoms which make the sufferers seek help. Whether in fact HRT should be started earlier to prevent bone loss is still the subject of controversy within the medical profession.

Although when HRT will be initiated is usually dependent upon menopausal symptoms first appearing in sufficient severity, the question of how long treatment should be continued will depend upon what strategy your doctor, preferably after discussing the various implications fully with you, will choose as most appropriate.

Essentially, the choice is between engaging in short- or medium-term treatment whose only purpose is to provide relief from menopausal symptoms or to choose instead a long-term strategy to provide, in addition, continuing protection against the risks of osteoporosis or cardiovascular disease.

If the initial choice is to provide HRT simply for symptom relief, then treatment will generally last two to three years. After that period, if the menopausal symptoms haven't recurred, treatment will be withdrawn. Should the menopausal symptoms reappear after treatment has been withdrawn, then it may be started again, probably on a year-to-year basis until the patient remains free of symptoms.

Although attitudes among doctors vary widely on this subject, most will generally prefer to prescribe HRT for symptom relief only and there is still a certain reluctance to provide treatment for *prophylaxis* – that is to 'prevent' – against osteoporosis and cardiovascular risks. The reason for this is that if HRT is to prevent these risks it will need to be taken for a much longer period and this means making a conscious decision to place the patient on an HRT regimen for at least five years and probably for ten years or even longer.

Considering the length of time that HRT is needed for prophylaxis, it is not surprising that many doctors prefer not to commit themselves to this course at the outset of the menopause and generally prefer to postpone the decision whether to continue treatment after the menopause until all its symptoms have disappeared.

Sometimes, however, it may be particularly appropriate to start long-term treatment right from the outset and there are certain cases where there is a strong enough indication that justifiable benefits will be derived from it. Patients who are likely candidates for long-term treatment include:

- Those women who have had symptomatic genital tract changes and these have been reversed by initial treatment.
- Patients who have had surgery for urinary incontinence or who have had prolapse repair.
- Patients who already have osteoporosis or coronary heart disease, as well as those where there is a family history of osteoporosis.
- Women who have had a premature menopause and therefore are much more at risk at a comparatively early age from both osteoporosis and cardiovascular problems. An indication of how greatly these risks increase under certain circumstances is shown by studies that estimated that the risk of myocardial infarction was four to five times higher for women who had experienced premature ovarian failure. As far as osteoporosis is concerned, premature ovarian failure will bring forward the age when this occurs and therefore the likelihood of fractures. And this means that – going on the generally accepted assumption that susceptible individuals reach their theoretical fracture threshold some 10 to 15 years after ovarian failure – women who became menopausal before the age of 40 will be at risk of fracture as early as their fifties.

Although this chapter has covered the main points of HRT and how it is used most commonly in the majority of cases, there are instances where special circumstances apply and the treatment may need to be modified accordingly. These special aspects of HRT are covered in the next chapter.

11 Special Aspects Of Hormone Replacement Therapy

Although for most women the provision of Hormone Replacement Therapy is a fairly straightforward matter nowadays and – subject to the guidelines covered in the previous chapter – is likely to cause few, if any, problems, there are instances where special care is needed to ensure that the treatment is both as safe and as efficient as possible.

PRE-EXISTING MEDICAL CONDITIONS

Treatment by HRT may need to be modified to match the special needs of patients who have certain pre-existing medical conditions.

DIABETES. There had been some concern within the medical profession in the past as to whether HRT was suitable for diabetic patients, as there had been reports of adverse effects on liver function and glucose tolerance.

Current thinking, however, suggests that there is no evidence that postmenopausal oestrogen replacement adversely affects carbohydrate metabolism and it is now accepted that there is no reason not to provide HRT for diabetic women. Nevertheless, if treatment is started, the patient's glycaemic control should be carefully monitored as the insulin dose may need to be altered as progestogens can have an anti-insulin effect.

There is also a reason why the use of HRT may be particularly indicated in these instances and this is because all diabetics are at greater risk from cardiovascular disease. HRT, as seen in the previous chapter, is cardioprotective and therefore reduces this risk. Diabetic women are also as a group at greater risk from emdometrial cancer and therefore it is important that progestogens are part of the HRT regimen.

PREVIOUS THROMBOEMBOLISM. Although until recently it was believed that a history of previous thromboembolism was a contra-indication to HRT, there is now some doubt about that view as it was based upon experience with the contraceptive pill. Current thinking suggests that HRT might still be suitable for patients with a history of thromboembolism, particularly if that was the result of a specific provoking incident, such as prolonged bed rest or surgery. However, if HRT is to be used, it is generally accepted that it should be in the form of implants, skin patches or vaginal creams rather than orally as these methods avoid the liver.

Additionally, it is generally recommended that special investigations – including screening for intrinsic prothrombotic tendency, antithrombin III, protein C deficiency, abnormal clotting and fibrinogen/platelet malfunction – should be undertaken before prescribing HRT for women who had an episode of thromboembolism either while taking the contraceptive pill or during pregnancy.

ENDOMETRIAL CANCER. There seems to be no hard and fast rules here and the decision as to whether to provide HRT should be made on an individual basis taking into account the extent to which the myometrium is affected and whether there is cervical or extra-uterine involvement.

GALLSTONES. Special care should be taken when considering HRT for a patient with a history of gallstones as both oral artificial oestrogens and natural oestrogens increase the risk of gallstones. To date, there is no data on whether oestrogen administered by transdermal patch creates the same effect and therefore that may be an alternative route of administration.

SMOKERS. Smoking, of course, is a major risk factor for myocardial infarction and stroke. While the use of oral contraceptives were shown to increase this risk there is no solid data to support the view that HRT would do the same. The current thinking is that HRT should not be withheld from women who smoke although they should be encouraged to give up the habit. It has also been found that oestrogen seems to have the same cardioprotective effect against heart attacks and stroke for women who smoke as for those who don't.

OTOSCLEROSIS. There is some question as to whether HRT should be used by women who suffer from this comparatively rare condition which is a deterioration of the inner part of the ear and can cause noises in the ear (*Tinnitus*) and gradually increasing deafness. As this condition has been seen frequently to deteriorate during pregnancy it has been linked to exogenous oestrogens and therefore it has been seen by some as a contra-indication to HRT. On the other hand, there is no solid data to show that HRT causes the condition to deteriorate.

VARIOUS GYNAECOLOGICAL CANCERS. HRT can still be considered for use by patients who have a history of vaginal, ovarian or cervical cancer, providing these diseases have been – or are being – effectively treated. To date, there is no evidence that oestrogen plays any role in increasing the risk of these cancers occurring.

WHAT SCREENING IS RECOMMENDED?

While HRT is well tolerated by most women, there is always a need to monitor the regimen and adjust it if necessary. For most patients – where there were no previous contra-indications – the following screening is generally considered to be sufficient.

Before HRT is started: cervical smear, pelvic examination, blood pressure and weight check, breast examination, mammogram and/or bone densimetry if available.

This should be followed up at least every six months by checking the weight and blood pressure and to these should be added every year, breast examination and pelvic examination if cervical cytology is needed. Additionally, mammography and pelvic examination should be carried out every three years.

The above, of course, are minimum recommendations for a screening programme and any unusual symptoms would require more frequent check-ups. Somewhat contrary to popular belief, there is no statistical evidence to support the suggestion that oestrogen significantly increases either weight or blood pressure (either systolic or diastolic). Nevertheless, the response to HRT varies considerably and weight gain or rising blood pressure has been noted to occur in some women after starting HRT and therefore it is advisable that both of these be checked at least twice a year.

POSSIBLE SIDE-EFFECTS OF HRT

Side-effects occur quite commonly during HRT and generally are caused by either too much or too little oestrogen or progestogen and the treatment may have to be adjusted accordingly.

The timing of the side-effects within the cycle will often provide a clue as to which of the two components is most likely to be responsible. If the side-effects persist throughout the cycle, then the chances are that the oestrogen dose will need adjustment. Should the side-effects only appear during the part of the cycle when progestogen is also provided, then it's very likely that it is this dosage which needs to be altered.

As a generality, it can be said that the incidence of hot flushes gives an excellent initial indication of whether the level of oestrogen is correctly prescribed for a particular patient. Should a woman continue to experience hot flushes after starting HRT, then it's likely that these symptoms will disappear if the oestrogen is increased. Other side-effects that are likely to be reduced by upping the oestrogen dose include: headaches, lethargy, insomnia, poor libido and formication – the latter being experiencing a sensation as though ants were crawling over the skin.

The symptoms that indicate the possibility of the initial dose of oestrogen being too high include heavy bleeding, fluid retention, nausea, and increased appetite. Generally these symptoms will disappear by reducing the oestrogen, although on most occasions they will also quite often disappear naturally within the first few weeks of treatment without adjusting the dosage.

Another side-effect that is reported by about ten per cent of women starting HRT is the occurrence of symptoms that can be best described as 'premenstrual-like' and include: feeling bloated, breast pain, irritability, aggressive attitudes, fluid retention, anxiety and/or depression. These premenstrual-like side-effects are almost certainly due to the progestogen part of the treatment and are therefore likely to respond best to either lowering the progestogen dose or changing its type.

Heavy bleeding is another quite common side-effect and relief is often obtained by reducing the oestrogen or increasing the progestogen – or by a combination of both of these measures.

Migraine attacks may also be part of the side-effects of HRT. When these occur they are likely to be due to either relative oestrogen deficiency or to the effects of the progestogen. Once again, the timing of the migraine attacks is likely to provide a clue as to which of these two possibilities is the more likely one. Should the migraines occur during the progestogen phase of the treatment cycle, then they may respond to one of three possible modifications to the regimen: increasing the oestrogen dose, or reducing the progestogen component, or using an alternative progestogen.

It's clear from the above that the mere appearance of unwanted side-effects does not necessarily mean that HRT should be discontinued and usually all that is required is an adjustment in the treatment. There is, however, anecdotal evidence to suggest that some women are reluctant to report side-effects fully as they fear that this may lead to HRT being withdrawn and that, all things considered, they prefer putting up with the side-effects rather than going back to how they felt before HRT. While this reaction may be understandable, it cannot be stressed too strongly that you should inform your doctor of any unusual symptoms you experience after beginning treatment. As stated earlier, in most cases all that will be needed to rectify the situation will be a minor adjustment to one or both of the components of your particular treatment.

THE OLDER POSTMENOPAUSAL WOMAN

Although HRT is generally prescribed to relieve the symptoms of the menopause itself – or to provide protection against other future risks – and therefore is usually supplied in the first instance to women aged in their forties and fifties, there is a growing demand for it by older women who are well past their menopause. Although these postmenopausal patients will be free of the menopausal symptoms themselves, HRT may still be indicated for treating certain continuing symptoms – such as vaginal atrophy, prolapse or urinary incontinence – as these can in many instances be reversed by HRT.

Although HRT may be beneficial to such patients, there is often a reluctance on their part to accept the renewed withdrawal bleeding which may happen. After having been free of periods for perhaps several years, it is not surprising that women in the older age group may resist a treatment which causes bleeding to reappear. However, the older the patient is, accordingly lessens the chance of bleeding occurring and many patients whose HRT was initiated when they were in their sixties do not experience bleeding.

If bleeding does happen – and is not acceptable to the patient – an alternative form of HRT consisting only of progestogen may be worth considering. For example, one such regimen – *norethisteron*, dose 5 mg daily – has been found to help preserve bone as well as relieve flushing. Although oestrogen continues to be the treatment of choice for established osteoporosis, there are also alternatives – such as *calcitonin* or *sodium etidronate* – which may help those who do not wish to experience withdrawal bleeding.

THE BREAST AND HORMONE REPLACEMENT THERAPY

The extent to which HRT may increase the long-term risks of breast cancer is still an area where the medical profession has been unable to reach a consensus so far.

There were several studies in the past which had indicated an increased risk of breast cancer in patients on HRT. However, since then, many of these findings have been countered on the grounds that the original studies contained methodological faults and had failed to fully take into account many important factors, such as the age at which periods had started, age at the menopause, and the length of time that treatment had been administered.

Further studies since then – these being considered to be better controlled – seem to indicate that there is a lack of adverse effect regarding breast cancer from the comparatively short-term use of HRT, short-term in this instance meaning up to seven years.

That, of course, still leaves somewhat open the question of risk for long-term treatment in excess of seven years. The most recent evidence available on this – based on four studies – is that there is a 1.47 times increase in risk after using HRT for 20 years. On the other hand, three other studies showed that there was no increased risk. So, it seems that the evidence will remain contradictory for some time yet. The situation is further confused by the fact that neither of the two sets of studies referred to above involved a large enough number of patients who had been long-term HRT users to provide a fully satisfactory statistical sample.

To sum it up, it seems that the increased risk of breast cancer by using HRT is negligible if treatment is less than seven years. There is, however, some evidence that there may be a possibility of increased risk of developing breast cancer if treatment is long-term.

As the evidence is far from clear-cut, the question as to whether to engage in long-term HRT is one that the patient and her doctor must consider carefully, taking into account the likely benefits of treatment as well as the possible, but by no means fully proven, additional risk of breast cancer.

There is one more factor that a patient and her doctor may wish to consider and that is that there is some evidence suggesting that women who do develop breast cancer may have a better prognosis if they are actually receiving HRT. Two American studies have shown that women with breast cancer and on HRT have a significantly lower mortality rate than non-users and that this decrease in mortality applies to both the age groups of 50 to 59 years and 60 years and older.

While the above has dealt with the chances of the risk of breast cancer being increased by HRT, it is, of course, useful to relate this information to the likelihood of this disease in general.

First of all, there are some groups who are at increased risk of developing breast cancer and these include women who:

1) Already have another cancer, and particularly so if it is of the uterus, colon or ovaries.
2) Are over the age of fifty and are still menstruating.
3) Either had no children or who were older than 30 years when they had their first child.
4) Have a close blood relative with a history of breast cancer.
5) Have experienced so-called 'benign breast change' – that is multiple small cysts with mild fibrous thickening of the surrounding tissue – a condition found in approximately one in three women of child-bearing age.

Although breast cancer is unfortunately all too common, causing some 15,000 deaths a year in the United Kingdom, it must also be kept in mind that only one in ten breast lumps will turn out to be cancerous and that only one woman out of twelve will actually be struck by the disease. The possible effect of HRT in increasing breast cancer risk must be seen in that context.

We will now look at some specific questions about breast problems and HRT.

Q. Is HRT advisable for patients with previous benign breast disease?

A. While a history of previous benign breast disease is by no means nowadays looked upon as an absolute contra-indication to HRT, the fact still remains that many family doctors will take this factor into consideration before prescribing treatment. Part of the problem is that, as is so often the case, there is a great deal of conflicting evidence. The situation is further confused because no one is even quite sure whether previous benign breast disease increases the risk of subsequent cancer – whether or not HRT is used.

Q. What about using HRT if the patient has a history of previous malignant breast cancer?

A. Broadly speaking, the medical profession agrees that HRT would be hazardous in this instance. However, some proponents of oestrogen treatment would argue that much of this viewpoint is based on what is only anecdotal data and that HRT might still be considered in special cases where both careful monitoring and good counselling are available.

Q. What should be done if breast abnormalities occur during HRT?

A. If the detected abnormality is a malignancy, it will usually mean that the administration of systemic oestrogens will be withdrawn, although – depending upon the individual circumstances – this may be a gradual withdrawal over a period of several months. Benign breast conditions, such as cysts, detected during treatment do not necessarily mean that HRT should be withdrawn, although should the condition be painful, the dosage of either oestrogen or progestogen may need to be reduced.

PREVENTION OF BREAST CANCER

Apart from the tests which are part of the recommended regular monitoring of patients on HRT, one of the most important measures that a woman can take to ensure early detection of any possible problems is to examine her breasts very carefully herself once a month. The importance of this self-examination cannot be over-stressed as it's clear that the chances of clearing up any problem that may occur are the greater the sooner it is detected and reported to your doctor.

The monthly self-examination should be carried out on the first day of the calendar month by women who no longer have periods – the reason for picking the first day is simply to act as a reminder that this needs to be done monthly. Women who are still having periods should, however, carry out the procedure within the first few days following the end of the period.

During the self-examination, you will essentially be doing two different things:

1) Looking for evidence of any irregularity, this including differences in the size of the breasts; one being lower than the other; changes in the skin of the breast, such as dimpling or puckering, changes in colour or texture; skin rashes; enlargement of glands in the armpits or near the collar bones; indrawing of a nipple or liquid seeping from it; over-prominent veins; and also swelling of the upper arm.
2) Feeling for lumps. This part of the self-examination is carried out by touch to reveal the existence of any lump or lumpy-feeling area.

There is a recommended procedure for carrying out the two stages of this examination, as detailed below.

Looking for irregularities:

1) After undressing to the waist, stand in front of a large enough mirror under good light. Carefully look at and observe each breast in turn, noting size and shape and keeping these in mind for the next time so you can spot any differences. You should also lift your breasts so that you can look underneath them.
2) Raise your hands and place them lightly behind your head. Once again observe each breast carefully as the stretch of your arms will emphasise any difference in size or shape. Turn sideways to the left and look again. Then repeat by turning to the right. Pay special attention to the nipples at this stage by looking for anything unusual such as excessive outward or upward thrust, as well as for signs of bleeding or weeping.
3) Stretch your hands gently above your head as though reaching for the ceiling and again observe each breast carefully in this position.
4) Place your hands firmly on the hips and press inwards

until the muscles in your chest tighten. Observe carefully again and, in particular, look for any puckering or dimpling of the skin.

Feeling for lumps:

1) Lie down on a flat surface with your head on a pillow and, ideally, with your shoulders slightly raised by a folded towel. Always feel with the flat of your fingers, using the pads of the middle three fingers which are kept straight. As you feel different areas, gently but firmly press the breast tissue towards the chest. Keep your left arm by your side and use your right arm to feel the left breast, moving your fingers all over its surface.
2) Press the breast – always in a gentle but firm manner – in towards the body. Make sure to feel every part this way by working in a spiral movement starting at the nipple.
3) Lift your left arm above your head and rest your head on it and repeat the same examination as above.
4) While still in the same position, finish by thoroughly feeling the part of the breast that leads to the armpit.
5) Repeat all four stages above for the right breast by feeling it with the fingers of the left hand.

Should you detect an irregularity of any kind – or a change since your last self-examination – you should report this to your doctor at once. Although most irregularities do not mean that cancer is present, it may take other tests for confirmation.

CONTRACEPTION AND HORMONE REPLACEMENT THERAPY

Although some might think that HRT – because of its similarity to certain birth control pills – could also fulfil the role of a contraceptive, this is something that has certainly not been adequately established and therefore should not be relied upon.

The average dose of oestrogen supplied as part of a typical HRT regimen is significantly lower than the doses used in the contraceptive pill to suppress ovarian function. So, while the oestrogen component of HRT might have a contraceptive effect, it certainly is by no means certain that this would be the case.

Therefore, it is essential that contraception – if wanted – should be continued by other means until the last menstrual period has occurred. In fact, the current recommendation is that contraceptive measures go on for at least one year beyond the time of the last period.

As a general rule, women become less fertile as they age and fertility starts a gradual decline from the age of about 30. However, complications with pregnancy increase dramatically over the age of 40 when something like 40 per cent of all conceptions are terminated. Although originally it was thought that the use of the contraceptive pill should be restricted to comparatively younger women, it is now accepted – following a recommendation to that effect in 1989 by the *American Food and Drug and Maternal Drug Advisory Committee* – that there is no reason to limit its use to an upper age limit for healthy women who don't smoke and who don't have specific cardiovascular risk factors. Additionally, it is expected that the development of new forms of delivery – other than oral – will further improve the safety of such treatment for older women.

A possible alternative which may be suitable for use by older women who do have cardiovascular risk factors is the progestogen-only contraceptive pill (known by its initials as 'POP'). This pill can be used up to the menopause and also has a good record in helping to control menopausal symptoms as well as those of a premenstrual type.

Two are two points which are worth bearing in mind when considering contraceptive methods in the later years leading up to the menopause:

1) The efficiency of intra-uterine contraceptive devices (known as IUCDs or the 'coil') and of barrier methods (such as diaphragms and sponges) increases in older women whose fertility is declining.

2) Natural family planning methods – such as those based on temperature or mucus evaluation to determine 'safe' periods for intercourse – become even less dependable in older women because of greater fluctuations in hormone levels.

Appendix A – Sources Of Help And Advice

The Amarant Trust, Grant House, 56-60 St John Street, London EC1M 4DT, is a registered charity set up to promote a better understanding of the menopause and to support and expand research in this field as well as make information and treatment available to many more women. It also operates telephone helplines (calls are charged at 36p a minute cheap rate and at 48p a minute at all other times) on various aspects of Hormone Replacement Therapy and the menopause. The numbers and the subjects covered are:

0338 400 190, Introduction and description of other lines.
0338 400 191, HRT – what it is and is it safe?
0338 400 192, When to start it and how long to stay on it.
0338 400 193, Is HRT suitable for everyone?
0338 400 194, What are the possible side-effects?
0338 400 195, How do I take it?
0338 400 196, Where can I get it?
0338 400 197, What checks and tests will be needed?
0338 400 198, What can it do for me and short-term benefits.
0338 400 199, Osteoporosis and other long-term benefits.

You can also write to them for a list of most specialist menopause and HRT clinics in the country.

British Pregnancy Advisory Services (BPAS), 7 Belgrave Road, London SW1V 1QB, 071-828 2484.

Central Council of Physical Recreation, Francis House, Francis Street, London SW1P 1DE, 071-828 3163.

Family Planning Association, 27-35 Mortimer Street, London W1N 7RJ, 071-636 7866.

The K-Y Information Service, 68 Oxford Street, London W1N 9LA, is an information service offering free leaflets on the subject of vaginal dryness to the general public as well as to the medical profession.

The Marie Stopes Clinic, Marie Stopes House, 108 Whitfield Street, London W1P 5RU, 071-388 0662.

Marriage Guidance London, 76a New Cavendish Street, London W1M 7LB, 071-580 1087.

National Osteoporosis Society, PO Box 10, Radstock, Bath BA3 3YB, 0761-432472.

Relate (formerly the National Marriage Guidance Council), Herbert Gray College, Little Church Street, Rugby, Warwickshire CV21 3AP, 0788-573 241.

SPOD (Association to aid the Sexual and Personal Relationships of People with Disabilities), 286 Camden Road, London N7 0BJ, 071-607 8851.

Well Woman Clinic, Palatine Centre, 63-65 Palatine Road, Withingdon, Manchester M20 9LJ, 061-434 3555.

Well Woman Clinic, Wythenshaw Health Care Centre, Stancliffe Road, Sharston, Manchester M22 4TR, 061-946 0065.

Women's Health and Reproductive Rights Information Centre, 52-54 Featherstone Street, London EC1Y 8RT, 071-251 6580.

Women's Health Concern, PO Box 1629, London W8 6AU, 071-938 3932. Please send SAE.

Women's Nationwide Cancer Control Campaign, Suna House, 128-130 Curtain Road, London EC2A 3AR, 071-729 4688.

MENOPAUSE CLINICS

There are National Health Service menopause clinics in several hospitals. You will usually need to be referred in the first instance by either your general practitioner or by another hospital. The hospitals with clinics are listed after the names of the towns in which they're situated:

Beckenham: Beckenham Hospital.

Birmingham: Birmingham Maternity Hospital Professorial Unit; Birmingham and Midland Hospital for Women.

Durham: Dryburn Hospital.

Glasgow: Glasgow Royal Infirmary; Stobhill Hospital; Glasgow Western Infirmary.

Kingston-upon-Hull: Hull Royal Infirmary.

Liverpool: Woman's Hospital Gynaecological Clinic; Royal Liverpool Hospital.

London: Dulwich Hospital; Guy's Hospital; King's College Hospital; Queen Charlotte's Hospital; Queen Mary's Hospital; Royal Free Hospital; St George's Hospital; St Thomas' Hospital.

Newcastle-upon-Tyne: Newcastle General Hospital.

Nottingham: Nottingham City Hospital.

Nuneaton: George Eliot Hospital.

Oldham: The Royal Oldham Hospital.

Rugby: Hospital of St Cross.

Sheffield: Northern General Hospital.

Stafford: Stafford District General Hospital.

Appendix B – Glossary

ACUTE	Of sudden onset (and possibly short course), sharp, also as distinct from 'chronic'.
ADENOMATOUS HYPERPLASIA	An abnormal overgrowth of the lining of the uterus.
ADENOMYOSIS	When fragments of uterine lining become embedded abnormally in the uterus wall.
ADRENAL GLANDS	Small glands located on top of the kidneys, which secrete 'adrenalin', a substance vital to good health.
ALVEOLI	Group of cells in the breast that secrete milk.
AMENORRHOEA	The absence of menstruation for a lengthy period of time.
ANDROGENS	Hormones that produce a masculinising effect.
ANDROSTANEDIONE	A product of the adrenal glands that is later converted into a weak form of oestrogen.
ANOVULATION	Lack of ovulation.
ANOVULATORY CYCLE	A menstrual cycle without ovulation.
ANTIBODY	A protein found in the body that neutralises invading organisms by binding itself to them.
ANTIGEN	A substance that stimulates the body's production of antibodies.

ANTI-PROSTAGLANDINS Drugs that may relieve menstrual cramps by their action in reducing the body's production of prostaglandins.

ARTERIOSCLEROSIS A hardening and narrowing of the arteries, usually occurring in the later half of life. Also occurs in younger people as a complication of various diseases, such as diabetes, hypertension and being overweight.

ATRESIA Disappearance of the follicles within the ovaries.

ATROPHY The wasting away or the reduction in size of an organ.

BACTERIA A general name for germs or bacilli of any kind.

BENIGN Not cancerous, as distinct from 'malignant'.

BIOPSY The surgical removal of a sample of tissue for pathological examination.

CANCER Cells reproducing abnormally within the body to create one or more malignant tumours.

CANDIDA ALBICANS A fungus that causes vaginal infection.

CARCINOMA A malignant growth occurring in any part of the body.

CARDIOVASCULAR Refers to the heart and blood vessels.

CERVICAL CANAL The channel within the cervix that links the vagina and the uterine cavity.

CERVICAL Pertaining to the neck of the womb (or the body when used in a different context).

CERVICAL DYSPLASIA Abnormal changes within the cells of the cervix. This condition is usually benign, but can be indicative of a precancerous state.

CERVICAL EROSION	A non-cancerous ulceration at the mouth of the womb.
CERVIX	The lowest part of the uterus which extends into the highest part of the vagina.
CHROMOSOMES	Structures which appear in the nucleus at cell division. They carry the genes which control the activity of the cells and the development of the entire organism.
CLIMACTERIC	The menopause in its broadest sense; the 'change of life'.
COLLAGEN	A substance that the body produces in the form of tough fibres and which provides strength and flexibility to many tissues.
COLPORRHAPHY	An operation that can improve bladder control by strengthening the pelvic floor if prolapse has occurred.
COLPOSCOPE	An instrument that provides a magnified view of the surface cells of the cervix.
CONJUGATED OESTROGENS	Oestrogens which are joined to other chemicals to make them more stable.
CONTRACEPTIVE	An item, preparation or method to prevent pregnancy.
CORPUS LUTEUM	Tissue that forms on the ovary after the rupture of the ovarian tissue.
CRYOSURGERY	The use of intense cold to destroy abnormal cells or tissue.
CYST	A smooth bag containing fluid or semi-solid material.
CYSTITIS	An inflammation of the urinary system which often causes a frequent desire to urinate with urgency and – at times – also with pain.

CYSTOCELE	The downward movement or bulging of the vagina.
D&C	Stands for 'dilation and curettage', a procedure during which the vagina is enlarged and a curette is used to scrape off tissue from the uterine cavity.
DISCHARGE	Unusual or abnormal secretion or seepage.
DNA	The abbreviation for deoxyribonucleic acid, a chemical present in all cells and which controls the activities of the cell.
DYSMENORRHOEA	Menstruation which is painful.
DYSPAREUNIA	Painful sexual intercourse.
ENDOCERVICAL	Within the channel that links the uterus and vagina.
ENDOCERVICAL GLANDS	Glands that produce mucus inside the cervical canal.
ENDOCRINE GLANDS AND/OR SYSTEM	A number of glands, such as the ovarian, thyroid and adrenal glands, which secrete chemicals (hormones) directly into the bloodstream.
ENDOMETRIUM	A mucous membrane that lines the uterine cavity.
FALLOPIAN TUBES	The two tubes leading from the ovaries to the womb.
FIBROADENOMA	A benign form of breast tumour.
FIBROSITIC BREAST DISEASE	A benign condition marked by small cysts and fibrous tissue within the breast.
FIBROIDS	Benign tumours.
FOLLICLE	A minute sac containing an egg.

GENE	A sequence of DNA molecules on a chromosome. The genes are the hereditary units which pass on through successive generations and determine the characteristics of the offspring.
GENITAL HERPES	An infection resulting from the herpes simplex virus.
GONADS	Can be used to describe either the female ovaries or the male testes.
HAEMORRHAGE	Bleeding, usually heavy and abnormal, either externally or internally.
HORMONE	The substance produced by an endocrine gland.
HYPERPLASIA	An increase in the number of cells.
HYSTERECTOMY	The operation for the removal of the womb (frequently the cervix is also removed).
INCONTINENCE	Failure of urinary control.
INFLAMMATION	The natural reaction of the body to either infection or injury. Usually causes pain, swelling, redness and heat.
INSOMNIA	Difficulties in getting off to sleep or staying asleep.
IRRADIATION	Using a radioactive substance – such as X-rays – to treat or diagnose disease.
LABIAL	Pertaining to the folds of flesh surrounding the external female genital organs.
LESION	Damage to a part of the body from injury or disease.
MALIGNANT	Cancerous, as opposed to 'benign'.
MAMMOGRAPHY	An X-ray of the breast.

MASTECTOMY	An operation to surgically remove a breast.
MENARCHE	When the first menstrual period occurred.
MENOPAUSE	When the last menstrual period occurred.
MENORRHAGIA	Excessive loss of blood during menstruation.
MENSES	The menstrual flow.
MENSTRUATION	The normal monthly bleeding from the uterus when caused by hormone changes.
MONILIA	Another name for the fungus Candida Albicans.
MUCOUS MEMBRANE	Soft and moist tissues that produce mucus.
MYOCARDIAL INFARCTION	Heart attack resulting from the interruption of circulation in the coronary arteries.
NODULE	A lump or mass, be it benign or malignant.
OESTROGEN	A hormone produced by the ovaries and which controls the female sexual characteristics.
OOPHORECTOMY	An operation to remove the ovaries.
OSTEOPOROSIS	Brittleness of bones.
OVARIES	The female sex glands.
OVUM	Egg.
PALPATE	To use touch and pressure to carry out an examination.
PATHOLOGY	The branch of medicine that deals with the causes of and the changes produced in the body by disease.
PITUITARY GLAND	One of the endocrine glands situated at the base of the brain.
POLYP (POLYPUS)	A grape-like tumour, generally non-cancerous, which can occur in the nose, ear, bowel or womb.

PREMENSTRUAL SYNDROME (PMS)	The various physical and psychological symptoms that are experienced by many women shortly before menstruation and sometimes for the first few days of the menstrual bleed.
PROGESTERONE	The hormone produced by the corpus luteum.
PROGNOSIS	A forecast of the likely course of a disease.
PROLAPSE	The moving down of an organ of the body and protrusion from its normal position.
PUBERTY	The age when the reproductive organs first become functionally active.
SALPINGITIS	Inflammation or infection of the Fallopian tubes.
SERUM	The liquid part of the blood; also an injection, usually produced from animal blood, used to cure or prevent disease.
STERILITY	The condition of being unable to conceive.
SYNDROME	A number of signs and symptoms typical of one disease.
SYSTEMIC	Affecting the whole body, as opposed to 'topical'.
TESTOSTERONE	The male sex hormone, small amounts of which are also present in women.
URETHRA	The passage that links the bladder to the outside of the body.
UTERUS	The womb.
VAGINA	The female genital passage leading from the womb to the outside.
VAGINITIS	Inflammation or infection of the vagina.
VULVA	The external part of the female sex organs.